DISCOVER THE LATEST BREAKTHROUGH
IN THE WELLNESS REVOLUTION

THE AMAZING POWER OF
STEM CELL
NUTRITION

HOW TO ENHANCE YOUR NATURAL
REPAIR SYSTEM **TODAY**

ALLAN C. SOMERSALL, PhD, MD

PHYSICIAN & AUTHOR OF 10 BESTSELLING WELLNESS BOOKS

The Amazing Power of STEM CELL NUTRITION

Written by Allan C. Somersall, PhD, MD

Published by The Natural Wellness Group

A Division of GE Publishers, Inc.

2-3415 Dixie Road, Suite: 538

Mississauga, Ontario L4Y 2B1

--

www.thenaturalwellnessgroup.com

Copyright © 2013 by The Natural Wellness Group

All rights reserved

ISBN 978-0-9810209-6-9

Library and Archives Canada Cataloguing in Publication

Somersall, Allan C. (Allan Calvin), 1949-

    Stem cell nutrition : how to enhance your natural healing system today / Allan C. Somersall.

Includes index.

    1. Nutrition. 2. Adult Stem cells. 3. Algae--Health aspects. 4. Nature, Healing power of. I. Natural Wellness Group II. Title.

QP141.S64 2013	613.2	C2013-901839-5

Manufactured and Printed in Canada

Cover Design by MargaretAanen

www.stemcellnutrition.com

The
Natural Wellness Group
the best of science & nature

What Other DOCTORS Say About Stem Cell Nutrition

"Dr Somersall has taken an incredibly complex subject and transformed it into a story that the reader can easily understand. What's more, he has done so in a way that makes the reader anxious to turn the next page to find out where the story goes. This is a great book for the lay reader, or any health professional who is still a little fuzzy about the intrinsic role of stem cells."

-Harv Haakonson, MD, FAOHM,
Physician, CEO Healthserv, Victoria, BC

"This is a thoughtful and insightful look into the role of stem cells and the surprising impact of unlikely natural products. It elevates the effective value of nutritional supplementation. Therefore it is a must read for anyone striving for optimum Health and Wellness."

-Dennis Forrester, MD, FCFP
Physician, Adjunct Clinical Professor, Mississauga, ON

"We are privileged to be living at a time in history when health, wellness and medicine have come together to promote true anti-aging. Dr Somersall is ahead of his time to write this book that any reader can understand and benefit from. He has brought together two new and dynamic fields – Stem Cell Research and Nutrition. It is one of a kind and should become a milestone in the wellness field during our time.

-Herman Bell, DO
Osteopathic Physician and Author, Inglewood, CA

"It was my privilege to have the opportunity to read and benefit from Dr. Somersall's latest book. Stem Cell Nutrition can become a great source of training for my patients and students. It provides a safe and effective solution for a well balanced lifestyle, including the support of the body's natural renewal system. I felt the author's cutting edge passion for natural health, good medicine and optimal wellness. You will too.

-Shahriar Vaziritabar MD
Physician and TV Personality, San Diego, CA

"To the contemporary patient who rightly yearns to play an active role in disease prevention and health restoration, Stem Cell Nutrition is a breath of fresh air. This riveting book shines a light on the underlying physiology that maintains and repairs our tissues on a constant basis. It illuminates the handle that any reader can utilize to take control. Loved it!"

-Mia Hosey, D.C., Chiropractic Physician, Melbourne, FL

Other Books by Dr. Allan Somersall

Your Very Good Health: 101 Healthy Lifestyle Choices

A Passion for Living: The Art of Real Success

Your Evolution to YES!

Understanding the Evolution of YES!

Evolutionary Tales by Dr. YES!

Breakthrough in Cell-Defense

Nature's Goldmine

The Enzyme Diet™

The Healing Power of [8]Sugars

Fresh Air for Life

DEDICATION

This book is dedicated to all the wellness pioneers who lived ahead of their time and so made possible for future generations to aspire and to experience, not just the absence of clinical illness, but rather, the best that life has to offer to each individual living in harmony with nature and science. As wellness advocates today, we stand squarely on their shoulders.

ACKNOWLEDGEMENTS

I am deeply indebted to a number of people whose invaluable contributions made this book possible:

To Don Karn who first piqued my interest in this subject and championed this project throughout.

To a number of editors whose diligence and care substantially improved the text. You know who you are.

To *Carolina*, my proficient agent of many years, whose expertise in all she does for all my books makes the writing more pleasure than work and makes each product a joyful prize.

To Margaret Aanen for an exceptional cover design.

To Harv Haakonson MD, Dennis Forrester MD, Herman Bell DO, Shahriar Vaziritabar MD, Mia Hosey DC and especially to Ambassador Ray Flynn for each of their kind and generous words of endorsement.

And most of all - to my dear wife, Virginia, whose patience and understanding has been a constant source of encouragement and support through the long hours of preparation. She is a skillful editor and a great sounding board for all my ideas before they see the light of day. Her love is unfathomable and her wisdom is invaluable.

To all of you, I am most grateful, for without such a competent support cast, this book would not become a reality. However, despite all these other contributions, in the end all the errors and shortcomings are mine.

Dr. Allan Somersall

Table of Contents

Preface

PART I
THE STEM CELL REVOLUTION

PREAMBLE TO PART ONE..9
CHAPTER 1 – STEM CELLS 101 – BASIC PROPERTIES
What exactly are Stem Cells?
Are there different kinds of Stem Cells?
Why all the initial fuss about Embryonic Stem Cells?
Can Adult Stem Cells deliver the same Benefits
Do Adult Stem Cells originate in the Bone Marrow?

CHAPTER 2 – THE NORMAL ACTIVITY OF STEM CELLS..............................25
The Stem Cell Theory of Renewal
Stem Cell Release from the Bone Marrow
Trafficking of Stem Cells
Recruiting of Stem Cells by Tissues
Migration of Stem Cells in Tissues
Proliferation of Stem Cells
Differentiation of Stem Cells
Natural Repair and Regeneration

CHAPTER 3 – THE POTENTIAL VALUE OF STEM CELLS..............................45
Stem Cell- Based Understanding
Stem Cell – Based Drug Testing
Stem Cell – Based Therapies

12-POINT SUMMARY OF PART ONE

PART II
THE EVOLUTION OF NUTRITION

PREAMBLE TO PART TWO..67
CHAPTER 4 – SUPPLEMENTATION 101: A REVIEW
The Food Chain – Why Supplements – Vitamins
Essential Fatty Acids – Herbals – Fiber - Antioxidants
Digestive Enzymes – Nutrient Delivery Systems
At the Leading Edge of Nutrition

CHAPTER 5 – GETTING TO THE LEADING EDGE...103
Algae sets The Stage
Enter Christian Drapeau
Enter Dr. Gitte S. Jensen
Enter Howard Newman
A new Hypothesis - Serendipity
Proving the Case

CHAPTER 6 – THE LEADING EDGE OF NUTRITION.....................................145
A New Wellness Strategy
Other SC Enhancers (Fucoidan, P. multiflorum, Synergy)
Release, Circulate, Migrate
Other Benefits of AFA (PEA/Mood, NK Modulation, Phycocyanin)

A 12 – POINT SUMMARY OF PART TWO

PART III
SOURCES OF INNOVATION

PREAMBLE TO PART THREE...179
CHAPTER 7 – FROM POND SCUM TO PURE GOLD
Basic Algology
Edible Seaweed   (*Poryphyra, Laminaria, Undaria pinnatifida*)
Microalgae as Food   (*Spirulina, Chlorella, Aphanizomenon flos-aquae*)

CHAPTER 8 – HARVESTING THE GOLD..209
A Habitat of Beauty
Algae on the Lake
Harvesting 'Golden Scum'
Processing of AFA

CHAPTER 9 – STANDARDS OF EXCELLENCE...225
Quality Assurance
Safety
Toxicity

12- POINT SUMMARY OF PART THREE

PART IV
THE WELLNESS TRANSFORMATION

PREAMBLE TO PART IV...243
CHAPTER 10 – NUTRITION AND MEDICINE
Origins –Discovery or Invention – Natural Intervention as Prevention – Health before Disease – Universal Application – Food Sources aren't Drugs – Biology or Biotechnology – Diagnostic Medicine, Holistic Nutrition – Not for Professionals Only

CHAPTER 11 – A STEM CELL LIFESTYLE....................................275
No Smoking – Managed Stress – Positive Mental Attitude – Moderate Exercise – Adequate Rest/Sleep – Complete and Balanced Nutrition

CHAPTER 12 – THE STEM CELL FUTURE....................................301
Unpredictable – Therapeutic – Limited – Problematic – Subordinate – Universal – Controversial – Here and Now

12- POINT SUMMARY OF PART FOUR

APPENDIX A...313

Preface

The stem cell revolution is here. Everybody knows that or at least hopes it's true. But who also knows that nutrition – and supplementation, in particular – can play a critical role, especially for those wise individuals whose focus is on prevention and the maintenance of good health and wellness. This book will demonstrate that surprising truth.

Indeed, with all the media focus and hype on the possibilities of regenerative medicine and potential relief for many who suffer with chronic and sometimes debilitating conditions, the public has been given exaggerated and somewhat unrealistic expectations. At best, such major breakthroughs are most likely decades away from any widespread application. At the same time, we have overlooked a much more pertinent development in our understanding of the role of adult stem cells in normal human physiology.

We now understand that stem cells constantly leave the bone marrow, circulate in the bloodstream and migrate into any tissue in need, where they then proliferate and differentiate to become cells of that particular tissue. This constitutes the normal renewal system of the body. In this book, we will phrase this reality in a convenient 5-point mantra: **Everybody has stem cells; everybody uses stem cells; everybody uses stem cells everyday; stem cells work ... and they work every time.** That's an amazing assertion with far-reaching implications and therefore, it is worthy of frequent repetition.

The second breakthrough discovery to be elucidated in this book is that certain natural substances can support this normal stem cell renewal process. That defines Stem Cell Nutrition. Careful published research has demonstrated that L-selectin blockers found in specific micro-algae and seaweed – namely, *Aphanizomenon flos-aquae* and *Undaria pinnatifida* – do enhance the release of adult stem cells from the bone marrow. Other natural substances complement these algae to provide support for the circulation of the stem cells and their migration into tissues in need. This book will describe these amazing developments in detail.

There are four parts to the book. The reader can choose to read them in any order for they are designed to be individually coherent and self-contained. For those less interested in the details, there is a Preamble to each part and a 12-Point Summary of each one for quick overview of the essentials. That could be for some more than adequate.

Part One describes the Stem Cell Revolution that has electrified the medical, scientific and wider community with the prospects of regenerative medicine. But after the introductory course on the basic properties given as Stem-Cells-101 in Chapter 1, the focus is re-set with the elaboration of the Stem Cell Theory of Renewal in Chapter 2. A whirlwind tour of the latest developments in stem cell science is briefly reviewed in Chapter 3, with the cell-based therapies (more appropriate for Stem Cell Medicine) reserved for the Appendix at the back of the book.

Part Two introduces the Evolution of Nutrition with a panoramic view in Chapter 4 of the developments in nutrition and supplementation leading up to the cutting edge today. That's where we find Stem Cell Nutrition. Chapter 5 justifies that assertion as it tells a fascinating yet true story of serendipity and how we got to this leading edge as three principal players take to center stage. The implications and applications of this remarkable breakthrough in health and wellness then follow in Chapter 6.

Part Three explores the Sources of Innovation as we take a trip in Chapter 7 to the US Northwest and the pristine lake region. There we find unique and surprising sources of AFA, blooming naturally and annually to provide a basis for the new Stem Cell Nutrition industry. It is there that we find out that 'pond scum turns to pure gold'. In Chapter 8 we describe the harvesting and processing of this nutritious 'gold', while in Chapter 9, the standards of excellence that guarantee quality and promote safety are reviewed in reassuring detail.

Finally, in Part Four we discuss the Wellness Transformation that Stem Cell Nutrition makes possible. Stem Cell Nutrition is contrasted with Stem Cell Medicine in Chapter 10 with a clear focus on personal responsibility, prevention, natural alternatives and an emphasis on the whole person. Chapter 11 looks into a possible Stem Cell Lifestyle that utilizes all the various wellness factors in tandem. Speculation about the possible Stem Cell Future remains necessarily vague and unpredictable in Chapter 12.

However, there is no doubt that Stem Cell Nutrition is an effective wellness solution for the present, limited only by personal lifestyle choice ... Read on!

Part 1

The STEM CELL Revolution

revolution: *a period or process of intense, fundamental and often rapid change, with major consequences for all concerned.*

Preamble to Part One

Wow! How things have changed.

I went through medical school at the University of Toronto in the 1980's. In those days, stem cells were nowhere near the research frontier as they are today. In fact, when you consider that much of the research being done today on stem cells actually grew out of the findings by scientists at my *Alma Mater* twenty years earlier, it is remarkable that the spotlight had not shifted to stem cells by then, not even there.

But then, **nothing happens before its time.**

Thirty years ago, stem cells were understood to be either (i) *germ cells* – male spermatozoa (sperm) and female *oocytes* (eggs) that combine in normal reproduction to produce entirely new, complete and independent offspring; (ii) simply undifferentiated *progenitor cells* that give rise to the various types of cells found in blood, bone and the lining of the gastrointestinal tract, or else, (iii) *primitive (tissue) cells*, suspended in their normal cycle but capable of proliferating when triggered to replace tissues on demand, such as in the liver, skin and endocrine organs.

Classic Histology textbooks at the time devoted very limited space to the discussion of stem cells per se and their role or importance in the maintenance of homeostasis. There was no mention of their value to normal organ or tissue renewal and the promotion of health and resilience on a daily basis. The prevailing dogma was that cells multiply (proliferate) and become more specialized (differentiated), but one process was usually at the expense of the other. It was believed that highly specialized cells, like nerve and muscle cells, did not multiply once they had matured. These tissues were therefore not being renewed, period.

Let's be more precise. The classic example is the adult central nervous system (CNS). Thirty years ago, all neurologists had bought into an idea attributed much earlier to the prominent histologist Ramon y Cajal (the Nobel Prize winner for Medicine, 1906):

"Once the development was ended, the founts of growth and regeneration of the axons and dendrites (in other words 'nerves') dried up irrevocably. In the adult centers, the nerve paths are something fixed, ended and immutable. Everything may die, nothing may be regenerated. It is for the science of the future to change, if possible, this harsh decree."

To put it simply, the doctrinaire position was that nerve cells did not –even could not – proliferate in the brain or spinal cord after birth. Just imagine how this misconception impeded progress in understanding and treating neurological diseases for decades. As we will see later, the truth is that neural stem cells do exist in the adult brain. In fact, the formation of new nerve cells has been repeatedly demonstrated and is now the basis of active research into treating diseases of the central nervous system.

But back to the eighties, where the focus was on blood cells and the variety of cell types that were found to be derived from hematopoietic (blood forming) stem cells. It had been recognized that these cells from the bone marrow remain poorly differentiated but are capable of extensive proliferation, persisting through life as a potential source of all the differentiated cells in peripheral blood. They also renew themselves so that their supply does not rapidly diminish.

The only practical application in those days – and it now seems so long ago – was the fairly common medical practice of *bone marrow transplantation*. This was a proven approach for treating some cancer patients. The standard use of radiation and/or chemotherapy destroyed unwanted cancer cells but also destroyed valuable blood cells and their stem cell precursors. So, prior to such harsh therapy, patients could be injected with drugs known to stimulate the release of stem cells from the bone marrow. Those blood stem cells could then be specifically tagged, isolated and later re-injected to restore the blood cell populations after radiation or chemotherapy.

Stem cells could also be extracted directly from the bone marrow in a large bone of a potential donor (typically from the pelvis), usually under general anesthesia. For small children, stem cells derived from umbilical cord blood has also been used. These treatments have not been without potential complications and therefore, they have generally been reserved for more serious and even life-threatening diseases.

Now fast-forward thirty years and the whole western world is abuzz with the miraculous prospects of stem cell applications. Today the media hype has stimulated public imagination to the extent that what was until recently nothing more than science fiction, has now become desperate hope and unrealistic expectation. Ordinary people dream of a new era of medicine in which deadly diseases will be "cured" with custom-made tissues and organs derived from wonder-working stem cells. If we could remove all limitations, put any ethical considerations aside and leave the researchers to exploit these new stem cell capabilities – so we are urged to believe – then we could soon find an elixir of *regenerative medicine* … 'the holy grail of modern biology.'

There is no doubt that a revolution is indeed underway. **Hundreds, if not thousands of research laboratories around the world are spending perhaps billions of dollars each year, rapidly advancing our growing understanding of the stem cell phenomenon and its applications.** No wonder the Committee in Stockholm has awarded two *Nobel prizes for Physiology or Medicine* in this very field within the past few years.

In 2007 the prize went to Mario Capecchi, Martin Evans and Oliver Smithies for their work on embryonic stem cells from mice, using gene-targeting strategies to produce genetically engineered mice (known as '*knockout mice*') for gene research.

Just five years later, in 2012, the prize was awarded to Shinya Yamanaha and John B. Gurdon for their ground breaking discoveries that **cells in the body can be reprogrammed into completely different kinds**. Their work reflected the mechanism behind animal cloning and offers a realistic alternative to using embryonic stem cells.

Professor Gurdon was able to show fifty years ago that cells, even when differentiated and specialized, retain their entire genetic make-up. In other words, all cells in the body carry the same genetic information. That may seem simple or apparent today but fifty years ago, that was a rather uncertain question and something very difficult to prove. Gurdon proved this point by using already specialized skin or intestinal cells from tadpoles to clone more tadpoles. Eventually, and building on Dr Gurdon's work, other researchers were able to clone whole animals, with *Dolly* the famous *sheep* being the prime example.

 Dr. Yamanaha further revolutionized our understanding of how cells and organisms develop. In 2006, he used a relatively simple recipe to control just a few specific genes and turned mouse skin cells back into primitive cells which could then be modified to differentiate into various kinds of mature cells.

In principle, these are indeed revolutionary discoveries. Cloning animals and reprogramming stem cells is mind boggling. If stem cells do develop into tissues like skin, bone, blood, nerves, muscles and so on, and if such primitive cells can be generated and controlled, ostensibly by human ingenuity, then in theory, we could renew, repair and rebuild parts of the body that become damaged, malfunction or just simply wear out. That's the inviting prospect of a new era in medical intervention and cure.

But ... no so fast. **Miracle cures are not just around the corner.**

Despite all the billions of research dollars, private and public, and despite all the media fanfare and political posturing, the evidence of practical stem cell therapies to date is still very limited. Even the International Society for Stem Cell Research has advocated modest caution. They are quick to point out that while there are hundreds of conditions that can purportedly be treated with stem cells, the treatments that have been shown to be beneficial are "extremely limited."[3] Much progress has been realized in research laboratories, but successes in the world of clinical medicine have been few and far between.

That's the evasive nature of science and at the same time, the elusive science of nature. To show great promise is rather very exciting but to experience slow progress is always more sobering. Yet we should continue to dream of the revolutionary possibilities that the exploitation of stem cell science affords. But while we pursue these slow and costly research endeavors, we ought not to be blinded to another reality that awaits the open mind. Just perhaps, in nature itself, we may find a simple solution to some of these challenges. **Could it be that just as food preceded medicine, so Stem Cell Nutrition can precede Stem Cell Medicine?** Or, to put it in other words, could it just be that in the area of stem cell applications, the effect of nutraceuticals might be realized long before the anticipated breakthroughs in pharmaceuticals and other types of therapeutics?

That is what we hope to demonstrate in this book. We shall describe how natural, plant-based food sources can enhance the release and support the movement of innate adult stem cells from human bone marrow, through the bloodstream and into tissue. We shall explore the value of increasing such stem cell trafficking – not in the future, but here and now. We shall underscore a common solution for ordinary people to experience extraordinary health benefits and a resurgence of wellness beyond their wildest expectations.

However, we must begin at the beginning.

This text is designed mainly for the lay reader, so we dare not presume. It's therefore 'back to basics' as we set out on this incredible journey that's all about Stem Cell Nutrition. *The basic properties* of stem cells will be explained in a short crash course - **Stem Cells 101** - in the first Chapter. That should be quite interesting, especially if you are new to this field. Then in Chapter 2, we go on to explore *the normal activity* of stem cells. That turns out to be very surprising. We'll conclude this first Part of the journey by reviewing briefly in Chapter 3, how researchers today are trying to exploit *the amazing properties* of stem cells. Now that could be exciting.

Enjoy the ride.

CHAPTER 1

Stem Cells 101:
Basic Properties

The human body is the masterpiece of all creation… and what a masterpiece it really is! Not only is it comprised of an estimated 50 – 100 trillion individual cells, but each and every cell is a wonder of wonders! I often say to myself: *"Let the astronomers and cosmologists probe the dark eons of space and time, beholding galaxies and supergalaxies comprised of unknown and perhaps inanimate forms of normal matter, dark matter and even anti- matter. Let them speculate on the origins and destiny of these oscillating enigmas in the universe. But I would rather choose to gaze in awe at a single human cell right before my very eyes beneath a microscope, in a test tube or even better yet, in a living, breathing organism."*

These tiny cells perform zillions of highly complex and intricate but extremely efficient chemical reactions each and every second. They constantly interact with their complicated and changing micro-environments while at the same time maintaining individual homeostasis. They go about their many complex duties with absolute precision and in some cases, reproduce after their own kind.

Most cells assume a very specialized role in the context of a well harmonized body and are said to be particularly *differentiated* for specific characteristics. For example, blood cells carry life-giving oxygen and deliver it on demand throughout the body; immune cells coordinate a defensive system that makes for normal and specific immunity against invading pathogens of all kinds; skin cells provide a barrier to the environment, adjust for fluid balance when necessary and help regulate body temperature; gastrointestinal cells are uniquely fitted to aid digestion and controlled absorption of nutrients from food; liver cells are highly specialized chemical factories for metabolism of nutrients and neutralization of toxins and drugs. We could go on to elucidate about two hundred different types of cells that all work in absolute harmony for the maintenance of good health and growth.

We now understand that of the trillions of cells in the human body, about 1.5 trillion reside in the bone marrow. Of these, about 150 million have unique properties that allow them to be characterized as **stem cells.** Although that term was first used in 1909 by a Russian histologist, Alexander Maksimov [1], many decades went by before the physiological reality and its implications would get the acceptance and research attention that they deserved.

But in the early sixties, Canadian researchers James Till and Ernest McCulloch were the first to prove unequivocally that bone marrow contained stem cells [2]. They initially exposed mice to high doses of radiation that completely killed their blood- and immune-forming systems. Then they injected some of these mice with normal bone marrow cells. The result was that only the mice that received the transplants survived; the mice that did not, died. In effect, the new bone marrow cells that were injected rebuilt the blood- and immune-forming systems of the former group of irradiated mice. This phenomenon later became the basis for clinical bone marrow transplantation in humans which was alluded to earlier.

More than twenty years later, researchers learned how to extract the inner cells from mouse blastocyst – the hollow ball of cells that forms within a few days following the fertilization of an egg cell [3]. They were then able to grow them *in vitro*, (that is, working in the laboratory - in this case, in a Petri dish with special suspense media). These cultures gave rise to cells that reproduced themselves (by proliferation), but they did not adopt any characteristics of specialized cells (no differentiation) until they were exposed to appropriate biochemical signals [4].

So by 1998, the revolution was well underway after the team of researchers led by James Thomson, a soft-spoken scientist at the University of Wisconsin, Madison reported that they had succeeded in removing cells from human embryos which were fertilized *in vitro* and obtained from fertility clinics, to establish **the world's first human embryonic stem cell line** [3]. It did not take long before promises were being made regarding the use of similar human embryonic stem cell lines to treat many degenerative diseases and to provide hopeful cures for devastating and debilitating conditions that have an otherwise poor prognosis. Thus, a new era in medical therapeutics had dawned. It was only a matter of time before we could possibly learn to repair and restore both tissue and function, by design and on demand.

As simple as that, a sensational phenomenon had begun, but not without controversy, for at the center of the watershed development was a human embryo. That initial ethical dilemma with all its moral, religious and political considerations, quickly overshadowed the promising developments taking place rather more quietly with adult *stem cells*.

Now, therefore, we must define some terms of reference.

Even a most basic introduction to *stem cells* would constitute a book by itself. Our explicit purpose here is to elucidate the current state of Stem Cell Nutrition, so we must be very selective in covering just the essentials about *stem cells* to get to the heart of our subject where nutrition makes a big difference. Therefore, just to cover the initial bases, we want only to answer at least a Top Five short list of questions.

1. **What exactly are Stem Cells?**

2   **Are there different kinds of Stem Cells?**

3   **Why all the initial fuss about Embryonic Stem Cells?**

4   **Can Adult Stem Cells deliver the same benefits?**

5   **Do Adult Stem Cells originate in the bone marrow?**

So let's get started.

1.   What exactly are Stem Cells?

The term *Stem Cells* refers to a group of cells in an organism that have two defining characteristics which distinguish them from other types of cells:

(i)   They have the capacity to reproduce themselves (*replicate*) for very long periods of time (often throughout the entire life cycle of the organism).

(ii)   They can, under certain conditions in the body (*in vivo*) or in the laboratory (*in vitro*), produce daughter cells that eventually become other specific types of cells by a process called *differentiation or specialization.*

Let's put it another way. Other cells in the body which are more specialized are known generally as *somatic cells*. These cells never differentiate into other types of cells – brain cells are brain cells and will always be; pancreatic cells are pancreatic cells and also will never become anything else. Furthermore, they will often not proliferate (or multiply) and certainly not indefinitely. These are examples of cells that are highly specialized and fully committed to what they are and what they do. By contrast, stem cells remain undifferentiated and unspecialized in function until they receive some signal that triggers them to transform either by replication or differentiation into some other type of cell which finally becomes committed to its new identity.

A simple working **definition of a *stem cell*** has therefore been derived as *a cell that can duplicate itself indefinitely and become eventually cells of any organ in the body.*

In practical terms, two other defining characteristics are often cited to justify the classification of 'stemness' and any given cell group or type can be formally demonstrated to be 'stem cells' if they can be shown to also do the following:

(iii)   Differentiate into cells that are characteristic of each of the three so-called *germ-layers* seen in early embryonic development, and

(iv)   Contribute to the formation of a *teratoma* – a conglomerate mass of cells that on examination, is a collection of different body tissues and organs.

2.   Are there different kinds of Stem Cells?

The answer is certainly, yes! Stem cells may be categorized either by their origin or their destiny. First, their origin: in this regard there are three significant types of stem cells to consider.

Embryonic stem cells were first isolated back in 1981 from early mouse embryos. The detailed study of the biology of these mouse stem cells eventually led (by 1998) to the discovery of an effective method to derive stem cells from human embryos and then to successfully grow or culture them *in vitro* in the laboratory. More precisely, the cells are extracted from the very early embryo, or blastula. Morphologically, these cells are taken from the inner cell mass just as the product of fertilization begins to adopt some three-dimensional identity. In the normal course of real life development, the blastula would implant in the uterine wall and continue growing. In this way, the cells in the blastula go on to differentiate to produce all the various types of cells found in the growing fetus. That's the *in vivo* process. But in the laboratory where embryonic stem cells are derived only from *in vitro fertilization*, extraction of these cells prevents them from being triggered to go through that specialization process. Instead, when they are grown properly, *in vitro,* they reproduce themselves indefinitely and never quite develop the unique characteristics of specialized cells, unless and until they are deliberately triggered to do so by external changes in their choice growth environment.

For completeness, we should mention that scientists have also isolated stem cells from the amniotic fluid surrounding the developing fetus, such as is regularly collected in routine amniocentesis. These amniotic fluid-derived stem cells (AFS) are not identical to embryonic stem cells, but they have been demonstrated to be self-renewing and pluripotent [5] – capable of becoming almost any cell-type.

The term *adult stem cells* (otherwise labelled 'non-embryonic' or 'somatic' or 'tissue' stem cells) by way of definition, is really a misnomer because they are found even in fetal tissues before birth. Beyond the normal implantation in the uterus, some cells persist that retain the fundamental characteristics of indefinite self renewal and can, when required, generate specific differentiated cells. As such, they are truly stem cells … adult stem cells. We now know that such adult stem cells are found in a wide variety of tissues. The best known and most studied are skin stem cells and blood-forming stem cells, but the ever growing list now includes stem cells of the liver, lungs, skeletal muscles and intestines, along with those of fatty tissue, the brain, heart muscle, blood vessels, tendons and even the olfactory epithelium lining the nostrils.

In 2006, a new breakthrough discovery was made. This was one of Nobel proportion that we referred to earlier. Researchers identified conditions that would allow even specialized adult cells to be genetically 'reprogrammed' [6]. By controlling just a few genes, they were able to cause normal (and already specialized) mouse skin cells to revert to primitive cells. These re-engineered primitive cells could then be cultured to grow and triggered to differentiate into other kinds of mature specialized cells. In other words, they had produced what are now called *induced pluripotent stem cells.* **(iPSCs)**

This skilful manipulation has provided a much better understanding of some of the key principles involved in stem cell activity and offers exciting possibilities for advances in the biotechnology of stem cells. Because iPSCs are products of human ingenuity and manipulation, rather than the normal spontaneous direction of nature (unless it turns out in some way to be nothing more or less than an imitation of the real thing), we will choose to defer the discussion of these iPSCs until later in Chapter 3.

That leads us to the second way of categorizing different types of stem cells, by virtue of their destiny. Again, there are three basic types:

The mother of all stem cells is the fertilized egg or germ cell. This ultimate stem cell obviously has the potential to produce any and every cell in the body, since it leads to the complete formation of an entirely new organism. The germ cell is then said to be ***totipotent*** (having all potential) which means that it has the capability, under the right circumstances, to become any cell type.

One step down, would be embryonic stem cells that can, under normal circumstances, become virtually any cell type except germ cells. They are then referred to as ***pluripotent*** stem cells, meaning they have an almost limitless potential to differentiate.

Take another step down and tissue-specific stem cells can differentiate into multiple lineages, but all related to the tissue involved. These are called ***multipotent*** stem cells. They also show less self-renewal capacity compared to the *pluripotent* stem cells. The best example might be the different progenitor cells of the blood which give rise on demand to the various types of B- and T – lymphocytes, as well as other cell lines.

Research in the field of adult stem cells is continuously making new discoveries and our goal here is not to be exhaustive with details that only interest the professionals who work in this area. At the risk of oversimplification, we are reporting only the important highlights to introduce this new frontier to the lay reader. If we chose to be more thorough, we could go on to specify the different types of adult stem cells that have been characterized: namely, marrow stromal cells, or mesenchymal stem cells (MSC), Hematopoietic Stem Cells (HSC) and a more recent type, not fully understood or lacking definitive consensus among different researchers and therefore referred to by a variety of names: Multipotent Adult Progenitior Cells (MAPC), Very Small Embryonic – Like Stem Cells (VSEL) or Blastomere-Like Stem Cells (BLSC).

This level of discussion is not pertinent here but suffice it to point out that the Mesenchynal Stem Cells in the bone marrow give rise to the tissue stem cells, i.e. they have been shown to differentiate into bone and fat cells [7]; tendons, ligament and other connective tissues [8], as well as neurons [9] and cells of the liver[10], lung[11], pancreas[12] and heart[13]. That list is not exhaustive. Also, as their name implies, Hematopoietic Stem Cells in the same bone marrow are the well-known precursors to the wide variety of blood cells (red and white) and platelets[14]. But again, to be more precise, these same HSC are now known to also differentiate in some circumstances into cells of the retina[15], heart muscle[16], pancreas[17], liver[18] as well as nerve cells[19] and epithelial cells[20]. Finally, the Very Small Embryonic-like Stem Cells have been shown to have very wide differentiating capacity[21].

It therefore becomes obvious that the general understanding of this class of adult stem cells continues to evolve, but the trend is to a wider and wider potential for doing what stem cells characteristically do: remain dormant until triggered to proliferate and differentiate into a wide variety of tissues.

3.   Why all the initial fuss about Embryonic Stem Cells?

Human embryonic stem cells were the first stem cells to be isolated and grown in a culture medium. It did not take long thereafter for many big questions to be asked and wild imaginative speculation to begin. After all, if stem cells could be harvested and made to develop into tissues like skin, blood, nerves, muscle or bone, surely they could become, in principle, a kind of repair kit for the body. That would usher in the new era of *Regenerative Medicine* – the previous domain of only science fiction writers. Perhaps simple injection of embryonic stem cells would now lead to dramatic health improvements, surpassing all expectations of the best of drug therapies.

Maybe we could learn to control the genes in embryonic stem cells and then use these cells to effectively replace or repair faulty genes in specialized organs to restore proper function. Even more enchanting was the prospect of making major inroads in serious intractable diseases - from neurodegenerative disorders like ALS, Alzheimer's and stroke, to endocrine disorders of the pancreas or thyroid gland, or to far reaching and prevalent ones like heart disease, cancer and others. The possibilities seemed endless and expectations ran very high. As well, the level of excitement in the medical and scientific community and the public at large was palpable.

Then reality set in. The research activity was first handicapped by the profound moral and ethical considerations, since there are entrenched positions among the general public regarding the true nature of any human embryo. If human life does begin at conception because the fertilized egg has the potential of becoming a full human being, then the idea of sacrificing human embryos – even if from IVF clinics outside any mother's uterus – would constitute at least an equivalent to abortion. And there the battle lines were drawn.

But that was not the only issue. Despite all the frenzy of initial research on human embryonic stem cells, no meaningful therapeutic breakthroughs have been realized after several years. Moreover, in real life situations there is the significant possibility of these ESCs growing out of control to develop tumors leading to extremely negative consequences. Notwithstanding, the advances made with adult stem cells have proved to be much more promising and effective. More recently, we have also had the breakthrough option of using the third category mentioned earlier, namely ***induced pluripotent* stem cells** to which the focus of research has obviously shifted.

Over time, the existing embryonic stem cell lines have continued to provide a critical basis for further research into the many factors controlling the origin and function of stem cells. For example, after years of experimentation, protocols have been developed to trigger embryonic stem cells to form specific cell types by new methods of directed differentiation.

4.   Can Adult Stem Cells deliver the same benefits?

The answer is 'YES, and more!'

Initially, adult stem cells were somewhat neglected by the research community at large because these stem cells were believed to have very limited therapeutic potential. At first they also proved difficult to grow and/or differentiate *in vitro* in the laboratory. But times have changed.

The truth turned out to be more surprising than the fiction. Dozens of research laboratories around the world have since proved that **adult stem cells do indeed have similar capabilities compared to their embryonic cousins.** When studied *in vivo* – in real living organisms and not Petri dishes – adult stem cells can surprisingly proliferate and differentiate into a wide variety of specialized cells as needed.   For example, when injected into brain tissue, they can become neurons or glial cells[22], or when exposed to liver tissue, they transform to produce liver cells[23], and so on.

These and many similar observations raise a number of challenging questions. What signals induce adult stem cells to form in the first place?   Why aren't they differentiated like other tissue cells? Assuming they remain dormant until they are activated by some trigger – be it injury or disease - what exactly could that trigger be?   Do adult stem cells reside in tissue to provide local repair when necessary? Do they routinely circulate? Do they have common origins, if not common destinies? Can they make differentiated cells for tissues other than their own tissues of origin?   Questions like these have many research laboratories working overtime and as we shall see later, much progress is being made.

5.   Do Adult Stem Cells originate in the Bone Marrow?

Again the answer is an unequivocal YES! Even back in the eighties, hematopoiesis (from the Greek: *hemato*, blood; *poiein*, to make) was a recurring theme. This relates to the critical process by which new blood cells are formed. Most kinds of blood cells are highly specialized and cannot divide. They have relatively short life spans and need to be continuously replaced in the circulation. They are derived from hematopoietic tissues: both myeloid and lymphoid. *Myeloid tissue*, or the red bone marrow (Greek: *Myelos*, marrow) is the producer of most types of blood cells (excluding mainly T- lymphocytes which differentiate in the thymus gland). *Lymphoid* or *lymphatic tissue* is characterized by an abundance of lymphocytes and is responsible for the immune defences of the body. But the lymphocytes do not originate there. The B- lymphocytes originate in the myeloid tissue and join the T- lymphocytes as they are subsequently incorporated into the lymphatic tissue where they ultimately belong.

Bone itself is a complex and fascinating structure, too elaborate for any adequate description to be given here. Suffice it to say, that the compact or cortical bone defines the hard visible shell that gives bone its associated strength, whereas the spongier core contains red and yellow marrow in numerous small cavities. The red marrow is bursting with hematopoietic activity and much, much more – while the yellow marrow essentially stores fat.

In younger children, bone marrow is essentially all of the red marrow type, but with normal growth and development, the yellow marrow progressively displaces red marrow in the shafts of the long bones of the limbs. Subsequently, in adults, red marrow is seen mainly in the pelvic bones, the skull, the vertebrae and ribs.

Again, recall the classic experiments by Till and McCullough at my *Alma Mater* back in the early sixties. They showed that stem cells in transplanted bone marrow can, by and large, regenerate a mouse's entire blood system. Thus, mice exposed to lethal radiation were demonstrated to survive when, and only when they were given the bone marrow transplant[2]. That established the bone marrow source of hematopoiesis.

That's the best known example of stem cells being derived from the bone marrow. Other studies have also demonstrated that stem cells from the bone marrow could go on to form connective tissue (bone, cartilage, ligaments and so on), as well as blood vessels and other endothelial structures[24].

But that's not all – by any means! It's amazing how science advances. It took a totally remote discovery to advance this important frontier. Two Americans and one Japanese scientist were awarded the Nobel Prize for Chemistry in 2008 for the discovery and development of the **green fluorescent protein, GFP**. This remarkable protein was first observed in the beautiful jelly fish, *Aequorea Victoria,* back in 1962[25]. Since then, it has become one of the most important tools used in contemporary bioscience. By using DNA technology, researchers now connect GFP to other interesting but otherwise invisible proteins. This glowing marker then allows them to watch the movements, positions and interactions of the tagged proteins.

In specific stem cell application, fluorescent stem cells were injected into irradiated animals after this latter treatment had killed all the stem cells in the animals' bodies. In time, fluorescent cells began to show up in different tissues.[26] What's more, when any specific tissue was injured by design … voila! The area of injury glowed like a 'hot spot' of fluorescence. The implications were obvious. New functional specialized cells were being formed in the injured areas and since they were fluorescent, they had to have been derived from the bone marrow. My former high school teacher would have concluded: *'quod erat demonstrandum'*. Therein was the proof. In the words of the eminent stem cell scientist Christian Drapeau: *'A process that until then had been virtually invisible suddenly became visible.'*

In a similar way, GFP- fluorescent tagging has been used to demonstrate that **adult stem cells derived from bone marrow have the amazing ability to become** *in vivo,* **cells of the skin, retina, muscle, liver, pancreas, lung, kidney and even the brain. And it all happens naturally!**

More on that will come later. For now, let's just make one more observation. The reader might wonder at this point, if the bone marrow would not, sooner or later, become depleted of stem cells. That would be a reasonable inference if stem cells divided in the normal symmetric fashion. Basically, when normal cells divide, the double helix of the DNA unravels and a copy of each strand is synthesized. The two daughter cells each get one original and one copy of each strand. However, when *stem cells* divide the daughters are different, such that one gets to keep the two original strands of DNA and stay in the bone marrow, while the other daughter gets two identical copies and exits the bone marrow. In this unique process, the number of stem cells in the bone marrow remains more or less constant, even though there is steady release of the 'daughter' *Adult Stem Cells* from the bone marrow.

It is estimated that there are typically about 1.5 trillion cells of all types in the bone marrow of an adult. Of these about 1 in 10,000 or 150 million are stem cells, and at the same time there are about 10 million stem cells in the peripheral circulation. That works out to between 200 to 5,000 or more stem cells per millilitre of blood, depending on the method of quantification that is used. A good average would be about 2500 cells per millilitre.

The picture that seems to have emerged is that adult stem cells are continuously circulated in the peripheral blood for some time, anywhere from a few minutes to a few hours. In their normal course, they seek out or are attracted to different organs and tissues in need of repair, whereupon they migrate into the affected tissues to proliferate and differentiate into specialized cells of that tissue. If they are not recruited for assistance in this way, they can simply return to the bone marrow.

That is **the normal ongoing activity of adult stem cells in the body** and that's the process we will aim to influence with nutrition. But we need to understand it much better and that's what we shall explore in the next Chapter.

CHAPTER 2

The Normal Activity
of Stem Cells

A s doctors and scientists we love to take credit. We develop new drugs, therapies and surgical procedures that make a huge impact on the prognosis of real people with all kinds of medical problems - from minor ailments like the common cold, right up to serious life-threatening diseases and conditions like cancer.

In emergency departments around the world, patients in acute crisis find relief and often benefit from life-saving interventions by dedicated doctors and nurses, applying the best of modern medicine to relieve pain, reduce complications and save lives. Therefore, the diligent researchers behind the scenes and committed medical staff on the front lines deserve the highest respect, recognition and gratitude for what they do with such outstanding dedication and skill, day in and day out.

But it will do us well to stand back at times to reflect on where the real solutions lie. Assuredly, **the most important changes we observe come from nature itself and not from human ingenuity and intervention.** This is especially true for 99 % of the population that is not in acute distress but rather always seeking to maintain good health or at least prevent or reduce the onset or progress of chronic degeneration and illness. This is daily life, where ordinary people are in pursuit of normal health and happiness between those doctors' visits and before any reason to go to the emergency room. But more often than not, we take for granted that which comes so naturally and silently. We usually enjoy the benefits of nature despite our insensitivity and at times, ingratitude.

Let's illustrate. Most drugs are taken orally. Now just imagine the role of normal physiology in absorbing, disseminating, metabolizing and disposing of any drug you might take. Nature must handle that chemical imposition with careful discrimination and effective application, protecting the body especially from all the unintended and unwanted consequences. Or think of a surgical suture that can only hold the normal separated skin in apposition but cannot join or heal a wound of any kind. Yet it is natural to wait and see the skin remodel itself before our very eyes, sometimes without even the trace of a scar. Or consider the massive trauma to which the body is exposed in long or complicated invasive surgical procedures, which the body is resilient enough to withstand by processes that make recovery possible. Think of natural immunity and how the body is protected from all the pathogens and insults to which we are exposed each and every day. The vast majority of human kind survived for several decades, even before and without antibiotics.

Enough said. The Oscar goes to nature every time. **The real key to life and health is normal human physiology at work,** usually before and often despite our best medical intentions and interventions.

Now think of Stem Cells. The revolution we have been alluding to seems to put the brilliant research of doctors and scientists right on to center stage. Stem Cells now seem like something we are engaged in, as if it's all about us. There is something we have to do to make this work. We must usher in a new era of regenerative medicine with all the possibilities for miraculous cures that have eluded the best medical minds until now. And perhaps we will - just perhaps - and hopefully so.

However, as appealing and challenging as the new explosion of stem cell research might be, could we be overlooking the real drama that is unfolding? Before our awareness and understanding of the potential of stem cells were even realized, and before all the inevitable breakthrough discoveries that have been made and will continue to be made, nature is already at work, utilizing stem cells all the time in an amazing process of renewal and healing. It is hard to believe that we have been unaware and therefore indifferent to this amazing fact for such a long time.

To put it simply, **everybody has stem cells; everybody uses stem cells; everybody uses stem cells everyday; stem cells work ... and they work every time.** There is a mantra worth remembering! This is not a new invention, it is only a discovery. We have only discovered in the past few decades the natural and normal activity of adult stem cells. That's what we want to elucidate in this chapter and then, in a subsequent chapter (and the Appendix) we will go on to show how scientists and medical practitioners are already putting the new and interesting knowledge of stem cells into practical use.

THE STEM CELL THEORY OF RENEWAL

It was that last clever observation about nature that led two distinguished stem cell researchers to advance a seminal hypothesis in 2002, regarding the normal process of internal tissue renewal. In their own words, Dr. Gitte S. Jensen of NIS Labs in Klamath Falls, Oregon and Christian Drapeau of Stemtech Interntional Inc., San Clemente, California, proposed that based on a review of the earlier literature, "In situ mobilization of stem cells from the bone marrow and their migration to various tissues is a normal physiological process of regeneration and repair." They also proposed that "therapeutic benefits can be generated with less invasive regimens than the removal and re-injection of stem cells, through the stimulation of normal stem cell migration."[1]

In practical terms, the **Stem Cell Theory of Renewal** affirms that **there is in humans (and other mammals) an innate phenomenon of regeneration whereby bone marrow stem cells would sense distant injury, exit the marrow and circulate to a target organ, migrate into the site of damage, and undergo tissue-specific differentiation, to promote structural and functional repair.** (Fig.1)

This represents a bold assertion and if the evidence did not clearly exist to support the hypothesis of Jensen and Drapeau, one would perhaps wish to dismiss the idea even now as simply being 'too good to be true.' The concept of normal, spontaneous internal renewal via stem cell mobilization represents a novel and amazing idea that is so fundamental to health and wellness, that one is definitely inclined to wonder why such a conclusion was so long in coming. Anyone interested in natural healing, complementary medicine, disease prevention or wellness, must appreciate the power of such ideas since we again perceive the overwhelming wisdom and beauty of nature at its consummate best. What we would now perceive is *'stem cells already at work, promoting and restoring health to humans even before we master new technology to any possible additional advantage'*. It is an ordinary process, thereby possibly allowing ordinary people to adopt whatever ordinary means (Nutrition first comes to mind … but later …) to gain perhaps extraordinary benefits from enhancing this natural stem cell renewal process.

But what is the proven evidence that this stem cell renewal process does have validity?

We referred earlier to the initial stem cell studies utilizing green flu-

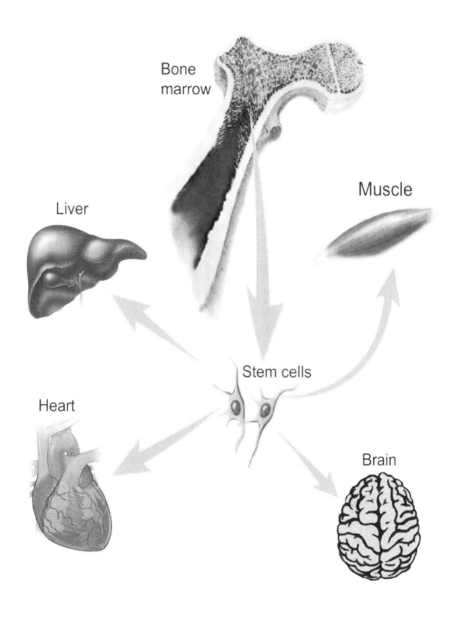

Fig. 1 The Stem Cell Renewal Process

Stem cells are released from the bone marrow, circulate in the blood stream and traffic to tissues in need. On arrival, they migrate out and then proliferate and differentiate to become new cells of the appropriate tissue.

orescent protein (GFP). As pointed out, when mice that had been irradiated to destroy their stem cells were then injected with GFP-tagged (fluorescent) bone marrow stem cells, significant amounts of fluorescence were seen in various tissues, especially in the areas wherever injuries were targeted[2].

The other classic study was done by a team led by Professor Diane Krause at the Stem Cell Laboratories at the Yale School of Medicine[3]. They used a novel technique known as *Fluorescence In-Situ Hybridization* (FISH). It's based essentially on exploiting the fact that males carry the X, Y chromosomes whereas females only carry X, X as a pair of sex chromosomes. The idea was to first inject an irradiated female mouse with bone marrow cells from a male mouse. By isolating a single cell from the bone marrow of the female recipient after 48 hours, one could then be fairly certain that it was a stem cell which would have the Y chromosome. When this was injected into a second irradiated mouse, it could, in principle, reconstitute the entire blood cell lineage all containing the Y chromosome. And that it did. Irradiated mice that were untreated survived for less than 12 weeks, whereas the second batch of irradiated mice that had each been treated with the Y-chromosome stem cell went on to live a normal life! That single cell (stem cell) was sufficient to rebuild all the usual red blood cells, lymphocytes and platelets.

That's amazing! But that was not all.

The researchers followed up the surviving batch of irradiated mice eleven months later. They must have been really surprised to find that cells from a wide variety of different tissues also showed positive for the Y-chromosome. They looked at lung tissues, the esophagus, stomach, small bowel, colon, liver and skin. They all contained Y-chromosome cells – up to 20% of cells in the lung.

Clearly then, the bone marrow cells were demonstrated to leave their home base in the bone marrow, to travel to the various tissues of the body, and then to become cells of those tissues. This process happened all naturally and spontaneously. Within a couple years, Jensen and Drapeau would formulate their insightful hypothesis that this represented the natural healing system of the body. Since then, numerous experimental studies have been published to not only confirm their hypothesis for consistency with known facts regarding stem cell physiology, but these studies have helped to elucidate significant details of the various steps involved in this critical process of renewal – a process that we will later show can surprisingly be affected by nutrition.

Let's examine the various sequential steps of this renewal process. It is very well described in the classic book by Christian Drapeau: *'Cracking the Stem Cell Code', 2nd Edition*, published by The Natural Wellness Group (2013). (This author is highly indebted to that source, especially in this chapter.) We begin with the release of stem cells from the bone marrow.

Step 1: Stem Cell Release from the Bone Marrow

I recall vividly in medical school how my perspective seemed to expand dramatically when I was first introduced to the structure and activity of bone. Those classes in histology were truly interesting. My previous thinking of bone was as a relatively hard structural mass, loaded with calcium but almost passive or inert, physiologically speaking. How wrong were those ideas.

The medullary cavity of each living bone is indeed a bustling factory with a myriad of full-time stem cell and other assembly lines, complemented by continuous input and output through a ubiquitous microcirculation of blood and lymph. The focus of this productive activity takes place in the bone marrow that resides in a seeming labyrinth of small spaces inside the spongy tissues that sit inside the hard bone cortex.

The stem cell assembly lines include the production and release of hematopoietic cells that give rise to almost all the blood cell lineages including red blood cells, immune system lymphocytes and platelets. They also, of course produce the so called mesenchymal stem cells or stromal stem cells that in turn leave the bone marrow destined for tissues in need of healing and repair, and sometimes eventually for growth of new tissue.

We now know at least three different compounds that naturally stimulate the release of these stem cells from the bone marrow: Granulocyte-Colony Stimulating Factor (G-CSF), stem cell factor (SCF) and interleukin -8 (IL-8). Of these, G-CSF has been most studied[4]. When first discovered in 1985, it was found to be a natural compound secreted by the body and shown to stimulate the proliferation and differentiation of granulocytes of the immune system. However, it was later found to also trigger the release of stem cells from the bone marrow and as such it became useful in application for cancer therapy. Prior to radiation therapy, G-CSF is injected for a few days to stimulate the release of stem cells which are then removed from the blood by flow-cytometry technique. The patient's stem cells are then frozen and later re-injected after the lethal radiation treatments. Like most drugs, injection with G-CSF does have side effects that would naturally limit its use.

Stem cell factor (SCF) is limited in any clinical application since it has been associated with rather severe allergic reactions[5]. Interleukin-8 (IL-8) produces a much more rapid release of stem cells (measured in hours, not in days) and has also found limited medical use[6].

For the 15-20% of selected cancer patients for whom G-CSF proves ineffective, a synthetic Canadian drug called Plerixafor (AMD 3100 with the trade name, Mozobil) has been approved for use when indicated as an adjuvant to enhance the stem cell release with G-CSF. What do we really know about the mechanism by which stem cells are released or otherwise, not released from bone marrow? Is there some natural control of this process?

The mechanism is known to involve chemical interactions between different external factors and specific receptors which are expressed on the surface of the stem cell. It does get a bit complicated but we'll try to simplify it as much as possible.

First, what makes the stem cells adhere to the bone marrow environment so they don't all go rushing off into the peripheral circulation? The bone marrow is constantly producing a substance known as Stromal-Derived-Factor-1 (SDF-1). This SDF-1 attaches to a specific receptor on the surface of the stem cells. It's called the CXCR4 receptor. When that binding takes place (formally described as the SDF-1 / CXCR4 Axis), the stem cell is stimulated to produce or express some special adhesion molecules on the surface called *integrins*, and these become the adhesive that binds or holds the stem cells in the bone marrow. So far, so good.

Now, as you would expect, anything that interrupts that binding mechanism just described would facilitate mobilization or release of the stem cells from the bone marrow. It is no surprise then to learn that G-CSF does disrupt the SDF-1 /CXCR4 axis. It activates several proteolytic enzymes that essentially inactivate or destroy SDF-1[7]. That does it. But G-CSF also increases interleukin -8 and how that affects the mechanism is not clear.

We just identified the action of G-CSF with the SDF-1 aspect of the SDF-1-/CXCR 4 axis. What about the CXCR4? Stem cells also have on their surface, a molecule known as L-selectin – a proven cell-adhesion molecule. This molecule turns out to be most remarkable in its own right. It is a protein commonly found on the surface of lymphocytes and interestingly on the pre-implantation embryo. L-Selectin acts as a homing receptor for some lymphocytes (mainly T-lymphs) to enter secondary lymphoid tissues via high endothelial venules[8]. In the pre-implantation embryo it acts as a receptor to facilitate the adhesion of the embryo to the site of invasion on the surface epithelium of the uterine endometrium[9]. Just think of that. It appears that in every pregnancy, when each and every human being is conceived, there is L-selectin playing a critical role, as the immature embryo gets attached inside the walls of its first home – the mother's uterus. It has recently been suggested that high expression of L-selectin on progenitor cells in the bone marrow is also a kind of priming for those cells being committed to becoming lymphocytes (on differentiation)[10].

Now, when L-selectiin is activated, it causes more CXCR4 receptors to appear on the surface of the stem cell. That would enhance the SDF-1/CXCR4 axis and further cause the stem cells to remain in the bone marrow. On the contrary, **if the L-selectin molecule can be blocked then the reverse will hold true and release of stem cells would be enhanced.** L-selectin is known to be activated by mechanical forces and/or by a ligand binding to a particular part of the same molecule. The important example here is that some sulphated glycans do bind to selectins to block them and therefore, they have been shown to trigger the release of stem cells from the bone marrow[11]. Now, just to tease the reader, note that some sulphated glycans can be nutritionally derived[12]. Therefore ... later.

Summing up, there is a natural mechanism in the body to release stem cells from the bone marrow. Upon any type of significant stress, tissues release G-CSF into the blood stream and upon reaching the bone marrow, it triggers stem cell release. That same type of mobilization can be affected by nutritional intervention, hence the title of this book is all about **Stem Cell Nutrition.** But there is more.

Step 2:   Trafficking of Stem Cells

Stem cells circulate in the blood stream. That's one thing. That's circulation. Stem cells leave the bone marrow and end up in different tissues. That's another thing. They're on a mission. They're responding to a summons, an injured or needy tissue has reason to recruit them. From source to destination, that's trafficking: leaving home, making haste and then getting to the destination, arriving at the goal.

What do we know about normal stem cell trafficking? We earlier pointed out that on average there are about 2500 stem cells per ml of peripheral blood. A reasonable physiological range would be about $10^2 - 10^4$ cells per ml. We know that individual values vary, with apparently higher populations during the day compared to night time. Younger people seem to mobilize stem cells generally more efficiently than older individuals, and women tend to surpass men. It also appears that the presence of more circulating stem cells facilitates the further release of more stem cells.

The stem cells appear to change during the course of their journey from the bone marrow to the tissues[13]. They have fewer adhesion molecules on their surface[14] and when mobilized with G-CSF as mentioned in the last section, there is an increased expression of CXCR4 receptors[15]. These same receptors respond to the SDF-1 (also produced by the injured tissues) which favors stem cell recruitment into those tissues upon arrival there. Moreover, specific enzymes that help penetrate the capillary walls inside the tissues are also increased in the circulating stem cells[16,17].

An interesting observation relates to the sedimentation rate of these stem cells. Generally those from the bone marrow tend to be smaller and show a faster sedimentation rate than those in circulation. However, when sulphated glycans are used to increase mobilization, the stem cells collected during the first 8 hours have the slower rate like those of the peripheral blood compartment. Yet after 8 hours, they show the faster rate akin to those of the bone marrow[18].Why? It's not clear at this stage, so there's obviously a lot more for us to learn.

Step 3: Recruitment of Stem Cells by Tissues

In any case, upon arrival at the injured tissue in need, the stem cells must be arrested there and then crossover from the circulation into the tissue involved. This process of extravasation is favoured in a specific area of the micro-vasculature. When blood crosses over from the very fine capillaries (which have smooth muscle walls and therefore significant blood pressure) to the tiny post-capillary venules (that have no smooth muscle), the cells experience a sudden drop in pressure. This triggers vortices that apply mechanical sheer forces to activate the same L-selectin we talked about earlier. The effect is the same, the L-selectin causes CXCR4 receptors to be expressed on the surface of the stem cell. At the same time, the injured tissue is secreting Stromal Derived Factors (SDF-1) and other factors that diffuse locally to the capillaries[19,20]. They bind to those CXCR4 receptors to trigger the similar expression of adhesion molecules that allow the stem cells to adhere to the capillary endothelial wall within the tissue[17,21,22]. Furthermore, the binding of the factors like SDF-1 triggers the release of enzymes to digest the lining and release the stem cells into the tissue matrix[7,23]. At this point, they have arrived to get their job done.

The release of SDF-1 by the injured tissue is obviously a key variable in this entire phenomenon. The effect is a chemotactic one, implying that the stem cells respond to a gradient of SDF-1 and go directly to its source. There is good evidence to suggest that several tissues naturally secrete SDF-1 constantly, including heart[24] and skeletal muscle[25], liver[26,27], brain[28-30] and kidney[31] – all very active organs. These are perhaps subject to minor injury on a steady basis and therefore require some level of renewal all the time. Moreover, SDF-1 secretion increases when particular damage takes place. This could be, for example, an acute heart attack;[32,33] reduced oxygenation of any tissue;[34,35] toxicity or injury to the liver[36,37] or a case of excessive bleeding[38]. The number of stem cells trafficking in the blood at the time of any such injury or need, becomes a key variable in the prognosis of any such patient conditions.

This is important. Heart attack victims with a higher number of circulating stem cells show better outcomes after six months, compared to those with fewer cells[39]. In a prospective study of over 500 patients with coronary artery disease, researchers established that low levels of circulating stem cells is indeed an independent predictor of major cardiovascular events, including death from such causes[40].

Factors that influence the number of circulating stem cells must therefore be of major concern. Of course, the possible impact of nutrition is our primary concern here, but other factors like cigarette smoking[41] and the use of cholesterol-lowering drugs[42] and steroids[43] are known influences on the same SDF-1/CXCR4 axis in tissues.

Step 4:   Migration of Stem Cells in Tissues

After stem cells have left the bone marrow, arrived at the injured tissues and emerged from inside the small capillary walls, they occupy the *extracellular matrix* of the tissues and must make their way to the specific site of injury or need in order to get their job done. That tissue matrix is comprised of a family of polysaccharides known as glycosaminoglycans (GAGS),which includes hyaluronic acid (HYA), as well as collagen, elastin, fibrillin, fibronectin and laminin.

Hyaluronic acid comprises the main infrastructure or scaffolding of the soft tissue matrix. On the surface of stem cells, there is another receptor molecule known as CD44 (one more example among the Cluster of Differentiation (CD) molecules seen on lymphocytes and stem cells). This CD44 molecule binds specifically to HYA which is also found on the capillary endothelium and helps to facilitate first the extravasation. When SDF-1 binds to CXCR4 at the capillary surface, the stem cells are stimulated to express more CD44 adhesion molecules and these bind to the HYA on the endothelium as extravasation takes place.

Now in the tissues, the SDF-1/CXCR4 activation also causes the stem cells to form pseudopodia (or literally, small feet) by extending the cell membrane directly towards the source of SDF-1 secretion at the specific site of injury. Again, this is a targeted chemotactic response. The same axis activation causes CD44 adhesion molecules to be expressed on the surface at the tip of the pseudopodia[44]. That CD44 binds to the HYA in the immediate environment, but the cell soon sheds the CD44 and moves along to the next available HYA in its path as it seems to just crawl along, using the pseudopodia as its small feet [45]. Amazing, but that's nature for you.

Step 5:   Proliferation of Stem Cells

The stem cells have arrived. At the point of injury in the tissues, they must now proliferate and differentiate into cells specific for each tissue. After all, we know that there are just not enough *circulating* stem cells to address the need for any significant injury or tissue degeneration. These newly arrived 'paramedic' cells must multiply and expand to get their job done effectively. And that they do. But these aspects of the overall renewal process require further study.

Despite the foregoing remark, there are some things we already know. The same SDF-1 has been shown to stimulate the proliferation and survival of stem cells under certain experimental conditions.[46,47] That's good and consistent, and may indicate that SDF-1 also serves as a 'cellular survival factor' in real tissues.[48,49] Also, insulin-like growth factor (IGF-1) combines with Epidermal Growth Factor (EGF) or Fibroblast Growth Factor -2 (FGF-2) to support the proliferation and survival of stem cells of nerves[50] and muscles[51]. Extracellular nucleotides (compare these with DNA building blocks) also support the proliferation of brain stem cells[52].

Lifestyle factors also play a role here. Again, nutrition is naturally at the top of our present list and evidence is increasing in this regard. Nutritional factors including green tea, catechin, carnosine and vitamin D3 have all been demonstrated to support the proliferation of human hematopoietic progenitor cells in culture[53]. There's hope for more.

The other relevant factors include sleep and stress management. The melatonin produced during sleep is known to enhance the proliferation of neural stem cells[54]. It was also shown to stimulate the release of G-CSF, which you recall, favors migration of stem cells from the bone marrow. How good is that? That's another justification for the value of rest and a good night's sleep. Among other things, sound sleep appears to support the ability of the body to rejuvenate and repair the nervous system. On the other hand, negative factors like stress and inordinate anxiety might reduce the ability of stem cells to proliferate. Again, we do have a lot to learn.

Step 6:   Differentiation of Stem Cells

Clearly, the stem cells from bone marrow respond to triggers from injured tissues and traffick directly to those tissues for the purpose of renewal.   Upon arrival they leave the tiny capillaries and migrate directly and purposefully to the action scene inside each relevant tissue. There they get down to business. They proliferate and then transform into a wide variety of specialized cells, specific for each tissue involved. There is clear evidence that these stem cells can differentiate into a long and growing list of tissues including:

Skeletal muscle[55,56] Gastro-intestinal epithelium[2,57] Hepatocytes[58] Pancreatic endocrine cells[59] Epithelial cells[2] Bone, [60] Skin[2] Neurons[61] Cartilage[60] Retinal cells[62] Endothelial cells[63] Lung[2] Cardiac muscle cells[64]

But again the question arises: What initiates this differentiation process in the tissues? How does the newly arrived pluripotent stem cell become sensitized to the local need to transform into cells of each specific tissue? Not surprising, the answer is neither obvious nor clear, leaving room for speculation and new hypotheses.

One proposed mechanism to trigger differentiation relates to possible fusion between each of the stem cells arriving as guest and a corresponding cell of the host tissue[65-67]. This 1:1 correspondence is probably inadequate and therefore unlikely to be a major mechanism, especially since cell fusion in real life is not very common. After all, cell membranes are designed to avoid such fusion[68]. But, when researchers at the University of Iowa recently studied cell fusion after bone marrow transplantation, they found that after cell fusion with embryonic stem cells, bone marrow cells were reprogrammed into new tetraploid pluripotent stem cells that successfully differentiated into beating cardiomyocytes (heart muscle cells). They concluded that cell fusion is ubiquitous after cellular transplants and that the subsequent sharing of genetic material affected cellular survival and function[69].

A more likely mechanism that has been proposed is that of induced or contact differentiation. In a classic experiment by Jang et al.,[70] hematopoietic stem cells were exposed in a culture medium to small pieces of damaged liver, separated by a semi permeable membrane.

This latter membrane had pores which were large enough to let ordinary molecules pass through but small enough to prevent the passage of actual cells from the compartment with the liver to the second compartment containing the stem cells. The results showed clearly, with appropriate markers, that the stem cells transformed into liver cells within several hours. This proved that differentiation is in fact triggered at least by molecules released from the damaged tissue getting into direct contact with the stem cells. No cellular fusion of any kind was necessary. Interesting, isn't it?

Even more fascinating was the course of differentiation. Different markers are found on developing liver cells in the young fetus compared to those in mature liver cells. Jang's team followed the progress of these markers only to find that during the differentiation process, the hematopoietic stem cell converts to the liver cell, all within no more than a day or two. That's awesome. And it is possible that the stem cells have a variety of surface receptors each of which reflects a specific type of ligand for each type of tissue as needed. This could then guide the type of tissue cell that results from the local differentiation process.

Further suggestion has been made that direct contact between the guest stem cell and a host tissue cell could provide a continuous function with some so-called 'tunnelling nanotubes' that form a cytoplasmic bridge just large enough to allow intercellular communication[71]. Of course that's possible, so research continues.

NATURAL REPAIR & REGENERATION

As we have seen, the detailed mechanism by which cells from the bone marrow are actively recruited to the various sites of tissue injury or degradation is slowly being elucidated through on-going research. Some aspects are much better understood than others but in real terms, scientists are getting a handle on this unique and fascinating healing mechanism. The entirely normal and natural renewal process can then be summarized as a product of **Six Key Steps,** briefly described as follows:

1. Release. This is the first and most important step. In the event of tissue injury or degeneration, specific compounds are secreted naturally to enhance the release of stem cells from the bone marrow.

2. Trafficking. The released stem cells are then attracted to the affected tissues in need by similar compounds that these tissues secrete.

3. Recruitment. Upon arrival at the injured tissue, stem cells have a facilitated extravasation through the small capillary walls.

4. Migration. The stem cells then migrate in a chemotactic response to a gradient of SPF-1 which takes them to the actual point of immediate need.

5. Proliferation. The stem cells have now arrived at their final destination and soon begin to multiply under the influence of a series of factors and influences in that specific local environment.

6. Differentiation. Finally, the pluripotent cells begin to differentiate into specialized cells of that tissue upon contact with its cells or signals from the extracellular matrix.

MISSION ACCOMPLISHED!

It cannot be emphasized enough that this is a normal process of nature. It has been taking place in humans and other animals long before there was any appreciation of its existence, any understanding of its mechanisms or any excitement and hype about its potential exploitation for therapeutic purposes. As technology advances we are prone to celebrate the great accomplishments achieved by innovative research endeavours everywhere. However, all the wisdom of the greatest research minds and all the acquired skills of the best human technologist would be better celebrated in humility. We must always acknowledge the vast intricacies of nature spontaneously at work, and how much more there is to explore and understand.

You might still be wondering if the renewal process described on these pages represents an actual on-going natural healing system of the human body whenever subjected to injury or degeneration. The answer is yes – **and this process is not confined to laboratories or to animal studies, but exists 24/7 with all real, live *homo sapiens.*** If that's still your concern, let's examine the results obtained from biopsies of sex-mismatched transplant recipients.

In an example of such cases, male patients were given liver transplants from female donors[72]. In some cases, unfortunate complications like hepatitis C and liver congestion necessitated regular biopsies to monitor the patients' progress. On examination, the tissue samples from the transplanted livers showed clearly the presence of Y-chromosomes. This was demonstrated in almost all cases and over a period of 4-13 months. Moreover, the relative population of Y-chromosome positive liver cells was found to be indicative of the patients' prognosis. Clearly there was effective migration of the recipient patient's own stem cells (XY) into the transplanted liver when damaged in post-op complications. This reflected nothing less than ongoing intrinsic attempts to heal the liver naturally.

Similar results could be presented for cases of other male patients who received heart transplants or lung transplants from female donors[73-75]. Again the evidence of Y-chromosomes in the transplanted organs leaves no doubt that the host patients were dispensing stem cells from the bone marrow to sites of injury in concerted attempts to repair damaged tissues, sometimes with actual evidence of limited benefit and success. Other biopsy results from later studies have also demonstrated that the same could be said of cells of the skin and digestive tract,[76] tubular epithelial cells of the kidney,[77] and even new neurons within the brain[78].

There should be no residual doubt today that in humans, despite the presence of local tissue stem cells that effect the most minute of repairs when necessary, **there is clearly an ongoing natural healing and renewal process involving the mobilization of stem cells from the bone marrow which are then directed purposefully to migrate into significantly injured tissues for proliferation and differentiation into cells of the affected tissue.**

That is nature's way!

However, all good scientific research aims to understand and harness the best of nature's principles and processes with the ultimate goal of exploiting them in the highest service of humankind. The same is true of stem cell research and that's what we will explore in the next chapter.

CHAPTER 3

The Potential Value
of Stem Cells

Thus far, our focus has been on describing the normal spontaneous healing system of nature in which ordinary pluripotent stem cells from the bone marrow are triggered by signals from injured or degenerate tissues to leave the bone marrow. They then travel to the site of injury and then migrate into the affected tissue to there proliferate and differentiate into new cells of that particular tissue. Again, we emphasize that this is entirely the normal activity of stem cells.

It's possible that because this is such a normal renewal process, it has not yet attracted great attention -much less excitement - either in the scientific community, the media or the general public. Instead, what has really captured the imagination in recent years is the possibility of human intervention and manipulation of these cells. In other words, the media spotlight and public interest has been exclusively on cell-based therapies, including the promising 'miracles' of *regenerative medicine*. Now the public dreams of rebuilding spinal cords for victims of spinal cord injuries in wheelchairs, or arresting and reversing the slow painful degeneration of patients with serious neurological conditions like Alzheimer's, Parkinson's, or ALS (Lou Gehrig's disease). We can imagine restoring malfunctioning endocrine organs that lead to diabetes or Grave's or Addison's disease, or rescuing dying tissues that would lead to cardiac or renal failure. What of reversing infertility on the one hand or slowing the aging process on the other? This is the new and promising revolutionary era of medicine that many now think is being ushered in on the horizon, thanks to stem cell research.

We cannot therefore leave this most introductory discussion of the stem cell revolution without outlining at least, where the state-of-the-art is in this area of research. We must consider what the prospects are for practically and realistically exploiting the potential value of stem cells, perhaps the hottest area of biotechnology in the world today.

Before we look into the latest advances and trends in scientific understanding and some of the anticipated therapeutic applications, it is again worth reminding ourselves that as simple as it may appear, **nutrition is still a major cornerstone to all health and wellness.** So in the end, we still want to come back to what nature affords in any likely food sources to benefit stem cell biology, even if that approach turns out to be relatively free and surprisingly easy. That we will do later.

For now, let's explore the potential value of stem cells. This is a vast and rapidly growing field of research, with new advances and breakthroughs being announced faster than we can digest them. Even what is reported today may be contradicted or superseded tomorrow by new discoveries. Therefore the information in this chapter should be considered not with respect to detail, but more importantly, in terms of the direction the work is going and the obvious challenges that are being encountered.

There is so much research activity into stem cells going on around the world that any attempt at a summary or update will inevitably be inadequate. Therefore this overview must of necessity be very selective and limited. As such, only some of the high points of recent discoveries and innovations will be presented.

There have indeed been some very impressive successes in the field of stem cell research. We shall try to outline these in three convenient areas:

1. **Understanding.** The development of stem cell science has opened new windows to investigate and understand many basic physiological mechanisms. Knowledge is power and therefore any insight into the natural order of things will prompt and guide new directions for biotechnology.

2. **Drug testing.** Stem cells are being used to derive what essentially are laboratory models of certain diseases. The responses of these prototypes to different drugs can provide a convenient alternative to the more standard animal models.

3. **Cell-based Therapy.** Here is the piece-de-resistance of stem cell applications. The possibilities of altering cells in the body or adding manipulated cells to the body, provide great opportunities for clinical medicine to treat a wide variety of diseases, especially some that as of now have poor debilitating prognoses.

STEM CELL-BASED UNDERSTANDING

Embryonic Stem Cells

Ever since James Thomson and his coworkers reported the isolation of the first human embryonic stem cell line at the University of Wisconsin in 1998, there has been an oscillating frenzy of hope and disappointment, success and failure. Putting all the ethical and even political considerations aside, the reality is that despite all the expectation from the public and premature claims from some independent professionals, there are as yet no approved clinical treatments using embryonic stem cells (ESC).

The only approval for any significant human trial given by the US Food and Drug Administration was in January, 2009. That trial was initiated in October, 2010 in Atlanta in the treatment of some spinal injury victims, but by November, 2011 the company conducting the trial made the announcement that it would discontinue further development of its stem cell programs. However, this decision was reportedly due only to financial reasons and not to any scientific or ethical considerations [1].

Nevertheless, all the continuing research on ESC has proved to be invaluable to the understanding of many of the fundamental principles of physiology with respect to stem cell properties and behavior. It laid the essential foundation for what was to follow and even today it still remains a very active area of research on many fronts. Scientists learned how to separate and culture; to stabilize and manipulate stem cells. For example, ESC lines can now be derived from a single cell taken from a pre-implantation embryo[2]. The cells can be cultured in a completely defined reproducible medium, using only human products. A wide variety of factors that affect the 'stemness' of ESCs have been extensively studied, leading to a better understanding of what's really essential and unique to stem cells in general.

Just to illustrate, and by way of background, consider the following. The DNA inside the cell nucleus is coiled or wrapped around some protein cores (histones) just like beads on a string. We have known since the 1950s that DNA governs protein synthesis. To make a given protein, the DNA around a particular histone begins to unravel or uncoil itself. On the other hand, that protein synthesis is blocked whenever the DNA cannot unravel. Genes for protein synthesis can become active or remain inactive by simply controlling the accessibility (i.e. coiled – uncoiled) to those genes. This is an example of a process known as *epigenetics*. That's the general term for the mechanism by which cells control which of their genes is turned "on" or "off", thereby determining the cell-function.

Now, researchers have studied ESC and discovered that simple methylation (the addition of a methyl group –CH3 to the histone core) can block some developmental genes. Elsewhere on the same histone, it can also prepare the DNA to uncoil[3]. These opposing patterns of methylation are called 'bivalent domains' and they allow the ESC to remain undifferentiated, while being ready to differentiate when needed. There are significant clues to understanding how stem cells can remain undifferentiated yet upon appropriate trigger, can somehow respond by initiating the process of transformation into a variety of different cell types, as we now know happens all the time.

Other researchers have looked at the influence of a group of proteins, called polycombs[4,5]. These block transcription factors that activate or turn on important ESC developmental genes. When they do so, they prevent ESC from differentiating. Other researchers noted that the same genes blocked by these polycombs were also bound by transcription factors known to be essential for the pluripotency of human ESC[6]. Hence, the same genes are, again, simultaneously blocked but still primed for activation. This is typical of the kind of understanding that is developing almost on a daily basis from the continuing investigation of embryonic stem cells.

Just one more example of the value of the ESC research should suffice. Neurodegenerative diseases are widespread. In general, scientists would love to find ways to adequately replace damaged or missing nerve cells with new ones created from stem cells. We know the latter are pluripotent and can form different cell types including nerve cells. But one of the major challenges is to determine how to grow stem cells into a specific cell type, such as neurons.

Researchers have studied mature neurons grown from at least two different human ESC lines[7]. They developed separate procedures to differentiate the two lines, first into neural progenitor cells and then into mature neurons. They used a new culture technique to observe the biology, genetics and development of nerve synapses (critical junctions between neurons that are essential for signaling and communication). They compared genetic microRNA's (which are tiny snippets of genetic material believed to be significant regulators of stem cell differentiation) produced by the two types of neurons. Both lines tended to produce different types of neurons but the factors that control why each hESC line produces a particular cell type still remain unclear. This type of work for example - illustrating why different ESC lines grow and differentiate in separate ways – promises to go a long way in helping others advance the biotechnology that hopefully can lead to innovation in regenerative medicine.

There are a limited number of laboratories that have utilized an earlier technique called *somatic-cell nuclear transfer* (SCNT) to create new embryonic stem cells. The method is conceptually simple. It involves taking the nucleus from a somatic (or tissue) cell from an organism and transferring it into an egg (i.e. germ cell) from which that nucleus has been removed. After being inserted into the egg, the lone (somatic-cell) nucleus is reprogrammed by the host egg cell. When stimulated, it will divide to form essentially a 'clone embryo' with DNA almost identical to the original organism.

An example of how this technique may be used for basic research is in the study of cancer[8]. Scientists transferred a mouse melanoma (skin cancer) cell nucleus into a mouse egg that had its own nucleus removed to then create a new embryo. Cells from this new SCNT-derived mESC were then injected into normal developing (host) mouse embryos. They found that these mESC contributed to different tissues in the host mice's developing bodies. In other words, the cancer cell nucleus seemed to produce normal stem cells showing that cancer is not always the inevitable fate of a cancerous cell. Yet the mice that were generated in this fashion proved to be more likely to develop subsequent tumors than normal mice. This is the type of work that can shed new light on how damaged or mutated genes that present in the nucleus of cancer cells actually cause the disease.

Although it was hoped that SCNT could be used to produce patient-specific stem cells to create new tissues for repairing damage or treating disease, the method proved to be very inefficient. Other methods have been found by using less-differentiated donor nuclei from neural stem cells in some cases,[9] and then on the other hand, by using more mature hematopoietic (blood forming) stem cells[10]. Those results remain inconsistent and uncertain. In fact, other studies of the early stages of genetic control demonstrated that the SCNT-derived mouse ESC were quite normal[11]. Another recent improvement involved creating the tissue-matched stem cells without cloning, i.e. using eggs from the demo mouse embryo that had been created by a process without fertilization by a sperm[12]. That technique has since been demonstrated for human embryonic stem cells[13].

Developments from this SCNT technique have not been without controversy. It sets some dangerous precedents with respect to the undesirable, unethical and to date forbidden possibility of human cloning. It is therefore now controlled by government authorities. However, in more recent times, it has become overshadowed by the latest exciting advancement with the reprogramming of adult tissue cells to produce induced progenitor cells that behave entirely like embryonic stem cells, even in humans.

Induced Progenitor Stem Cells

Fifty years ago, Professor Gurdon (the Nobel Laureate), had taken the DNA from specialized cells of tadpoles and cloned more tadpoles, demonstrating unequivocally that cells retain all their DNA even after they become specialized as in skin, intestine or brain cells. The challenge was obvious. Could such adult or mature cells be reprogrammed to function as stem cells which could again proliferate indefinitely and differentiate when called upon to do so?

By 2005, initial results showed that even human embryonic cells could indeed reprogram adult cells by fusing with them. But that produced tetraploids – cells containing four copies of the cellular DNA rather than the normal two. That obviously had limited utility or application. However, it was not long after, in 2006, that Shinya Yamanaha (the other recent Nobel Laureate) and his coworkers made the dramatic breakthrough[14]. They found that they could reprogram adult mouse skin cells by engineering the cells to express four defined factors: Oct 3/4, Sox2, c-Myc and Klf4, and growing the cells using embryonic stem cell (ESC) culture conditions. Those four factors are known to be important for maintaining the 'stemness' of ESC. As surprisingly simple as that ... the deed was done.

The new '*induced pluripotent stem*" (iPS) cells, as they were labeled, demonstrated the important characteristics of earlier embryonic stem cells (ESC). They expressed the same stem cell markers, formed tumors from all three germ layers as described earlier and they were able to contribute new differentiated cells to various tissues when injected into mouse embryos at a very early stage of development.

By the following year, the same Japanese laboratory was able to demonstrate the same remarkable results using adult human skin cells under similar conditions[15]. The laboratory of James Thompson in Wisconsin reported almost simultaneously the same observations with adult human skin cells but with forced expression of slightly different factors: Oct4, S0X2, NANOG and LIN28. Again, these gene factors were all chosen for their known importance in maintaining the 'stemness' properties of stem cells[16].

Those results opened the flood gates of research. First, the technique needed to be improved. The original iPS cells could not make sperm and egg cells when injected into an early mouse blastocyst. Now, with modification of the technique in mice, the iPS cells can make such germ cells[17]. When injected, the blastocysts produce all cell types within the developing embryos to the point where they can complete gestation and be born alive.

However, two major challenges remained before any possibility of transplantation in humans could be contemplated. First, the factors used in reprogramming included some cancer-promoting genes. In addition, the technique used inactivated viruses to carry the factors into the adult cells and such viruses can randomly integrate into the DNA host, which introduced the possibility that the virus would interrupt or otherwise damage a critical gene.

To address these major issues, some Harvard researchers added a potent chemical called valproic acid to newly formed skin (or fibroblast) cells in culture to help unravel the DNA[18]. This permitted access to genes as we described earlier. They could then eliminate two of the factors, c-Myc and KIF4, which are known to be potent cancer-promoting genes.

German scientists also identified adult neural stem cells that already express high levels of two factors known to be similarly important for reprogramming[19]. Using these starting cells, they were also able to produce iPS cells by inserting fewer factors – another step in the right direction.

The work of K. Hochedlinger and colleagues developed a special virus that allowed the iPS cell technique to be further controlled[20]. This virus allowed them to 'start' and 'stop' at will the expression of the genes used in reprogramming. With this 'on/off switch', they were able to determine the minimum amount of time that an adult cell must be exposed to these gene products in order to be reprogrammed. They were able to identify specific events such as the changes in level of gene expression or gene activation/deactivation that characterize the iPS cells at different stages of the reprogramming process.

Ideally, before any human application, the iPS cells would have to be generated and grown without exposure to any viral particles or any of the animal products used in standard cell culture media. Already this has been substantially achieved in the laboratory and the resulting iPS cell products have demonstrated the expected characteristics of pluripotent cells[21].

Scientists have also managed to reprogram mouse and human fibroblasts without using potentially dangerous viruses. In their advanced technique, the reprogramming genes and an inducible transcription factor (that is one which can be used to turn gene expression 'on' and 'off') were carried into the cells by naked DNA sequences[22]. In a further development, they also included with those DNA carriers certain marking sequences that could be targeted and 'cut out' by specific enzymes. The efficiency and safety of the technique were then markedly improved[23].

At a Massachusetts laboratory, researchers developed a novel reprogramming method that uses RNA to coax cells to make four transcription factor proteins that are critical for the process[24]. That made the formation of iPS cells two orders of magnitude more efficient and cut the time down from the standard month to a mere two weeks. The RNA finally degraded to eliminate the possibility of interference with the new cell function. The researchers used a similar RNA method to coax the iPS cells to differentiate into muscle cells by inserting RNA that encodes for muscle genes. That was another brilliant step forward.

Careful genetic analysis comparing the human iPS cells with embryonic stem cells and adult pluripotent cells show major similarity but with some minor differences that are not inconsequential[25]. They could possibly limit the potential use of iPS cells and so are being actively explored further.

Some Israeli scientists have determined that human iPS cells have chromosome abnormalities similar to those also seen in human embryonic stem cells[26]. For example, trisomy 21 (having three copies of chromosome 21, instead of the normal two) is quite common in each case. Some abnormalities arise through reprogramming itself, some through adaptation while long-standing in culture and some reflect abnormality in the original adult cell. In any case, one cannot be rushing to human clinical applications too soon. The risk of cancer (which is caused by loss of control of cell division) remains much too high.

In Canada, scientists have gone a step further. They were able to directly reprogram cells from one mature (differentiated) state to another[27]. They took human skin cells and grew them in culture with the addition of specific transcription factors (cell proteins that regulate gene's activity). These factors were again known to be important for generating blood cell types. And that's what they got. They formed new blood cells directly without going through or going back to iPS cells en route.

It's interesting that iPS cells do retain some bias toward differentiating into the tissue type from which they originated. A blood cell, for example, when used to generate an iPS cell, retains molecular markers of its identity as a blood cell, so it then differentiates (as an iPS cell) into a different blood cell in preference, compared to another cell type like a muscle or bone cell[28]. The bias can be removed however, by first programming into the particular cell type of interest and then reprogramming it for a second time.

There is still no rush to judgment or haste to human application of iPS cells because considerable problems remain. The fear of rejection and the threat of cancer are obvious limitations. In fact, in a most recent study, researchers showed that attempts to transplant iPS cells generated from mouse skin cells back into the same mouse were rejected by the latter, even though embryonic stem cells from an unrelated mouse were well tolerated[29]. This just highlights the kind of challenges remaining before any safe and reliable human application is forthcoming, as exciting and attractive as that possibility continues to be.

STEM-CELL BASED DRUG TESTING

In the normal course of research, understanding the basic disease mechanisms often guides the development and testing of possible new drugs for treatment of those conditions. As the underlying physiology is better understood, especially at molecular levels, hypotheses are developed for alternatives in therapeutic interventions. When new drug formulas are synthesized or isolated from natural sources, they are generally tested on small laboratory animals. Success at that level can then justify different early phases of human trials, and only when it appears sufficiently safe to do so.

The recent advances in stem cell science have now afforded new alternatives for this pathway of drug development and testing. We are learning more and more about the basic physiology of cells (in normal healthy animals) and in turn, about pathophysiology (the faulty mechanisms leading to disease). For example, we are gaining insight about the factors that control the on/off switching of genes that control protein synthesis (and therefore cell properties and behavior). This will go a long way to identifying possible drugs related to cancer prevention and treatment. After all, one could consider cancer to be, in the final analysis, the result of genes out of control.

Then there is the issue of inherited genetic disorders. Scientists have found during the course of *in vitro* fertilization procedures, that genetic diagnosis revealed that some embryos show evidence of mutation prior to implantation which normally mitigates against their use. Some of these embryos have been used to derive human embryonic stem cell (hESC) lines with different genetic abnormalities[30]. Today this provides an unlimited source of disease cells in culture that is being used to undertake further research on the primary disturbances of the on-going cellular processes in genetically abnormal cells. The current repository of these cells contains at least 18 such hESC lines with genetic disorders, including muscular dystrophy, Marfan's syndrome, Huntington's disease, neurofibromatosis, thalassemia and more. Such hESC lines provide an exceptional tool for study of these disease conditions and most likely, the development of possible approaches to both prevention and treatment.

With the advances that have made it possible to derive induced pluripotent stem (iPS) cells from individuals with known hereditary diseases, researchers have been able to generate cells and tissues for further study of the causes and possible treatment of such diseases, other conditions being equal.

The first case, reported in 2008, was of a patient with Lou Gehrig's disease (ALS)[31]. Scientists took skin cells from the patient, used viruses (as described briefly in the previous section) to insert factors to reprogram those adult skin cells into iPS cells and then generated a new ALS- iPS cell line. They could then coax these latter cells into becoming the type of motor neurons known to be destroyed in ALS. These new cells reprogrammed with ALS genes provide extreme potential for further study of the ALS disease process and for testing possible ALS drugs on human cells in the laboratory, before any human trials are necessarily undertaken.

Very soon after that report, other scientists reported similar results, generating new iPS cell lines that carry genes for 10 additional diseases:[32]

Duchenne muscular dystrophy

Becker muscular dystrophy

Parkinson's disease

Huntington's disease

Down's syndrome

ADA severe combined immune-deficiency

S-B-D Syndrome

Goucher's disease

Juvenile- onset (Type 1) Diabetes

Lesch-Nyham Syndrome

All these new iPSC-derived cell lines are certainly capable of long-term self-renewal in culture. This therefore provides a potentially endless supply of material for study of these types of disease processes and the initial testing of any potential drugs. However, the caveat is that the relevant cell types derived from these iPSC lines must of necessity be shown to manifest the associated disease characteristics and symptoms that would be expected. This latter concern has been demonstrated to be unfounded, at least in the case of spinal muscular atrophy (SMA)[33]. It is actually a group of hereditary diseases (rather than a single entity) that causes weakness and wasting of the voluntary muscles of the arms and legs of some infants and small children. Scientists were able to generate an iPS cell line from a child with SMA, and from the child's mother who did not have SMA. They found that motor neurons derived from the child's cell line began to die after a month in culture, but the mother's survived. Similarly, the same child's iPSC- derived neurons responded to treatment with drugs known to increase the production of the missing motor neuron protein. Therefore, at least in this case, the iPSC derived motor neurons exhibit important characteristics of the SMA disease. That's encouraging.

Studies of autism present another example of the same thing. Autism is really a spectrum of disorders. One of these disorders, seen exclusively in girls, is characterised as Rett syndrome (RTT) and is known to result from a defective gene. Researchers used skin cells from individuals with and without RTT to generate a new iPS cell line[34]. They then used that to generate nerve cells, which were shown to be smaller and had fewer physical connections (synapses) with neighbouring neurons, compared to similar normal neurons. More importantly here, they tested two drugs that are known to improve symptoms of RTT (at least in a mouse model) only to find that the same drugs improved the function of the human RTT – iPSC – derived neurons.

A similar result was found for Timothy syndrome which causes affected individuals to have irregular heartbeat, hypoglycaemia and developmental delay, and in more than 60% of cases, symptoms are consistent with autism. These symptoms are caused by an inherited change to a single gene. Researchers used skin cells from individuals with and without Timothy to produce iPS cells which were then coaxed into generating nerve cells (TS-neurons). These TS-neurons were again shown to have several abnormal characteristics as expected, but even more importantly here, they were able to identify a drug that can reverse these characteristics in the laboratory[35].

Other examples of the same procedure using iPS cell lines have been reported for conditions as relatively widespread as schizophrenia[36] (affecting about 1 in 300 individuals somehow, sometime) or as rare as gyrate atrophy[37] (leading to progressive loss of vision) or dyskeratosis congenita (another rare condition with characteristic abnormally-shaped fingernails and toenails).

What's the bottom line? Researchers are now actively generating iPS cell lines from individuals with a wide variety of diseases, particularly inherited diseases, and using these cells to gain better understanding of both the causes and any possible treatments for these conditions. Those are very hopeful signs for the future.

What is even more promising is the potential use of stem cells to develop cell-based therapies for a much wider set of even more prevalent conditions to reduce even more morbidity and suffering.

STEM CELL – BASED THERAPIES

Perhaps no other application of stem cell science has excited both the professional research community and the public at large as the prospect of exploiting stem cells for dramatic advances in the treatment of widespread major diseases and even traumatic injury. Unfortunately, and no thanks to all the media reports with hyped exaggeration, the public in the West has held on to immediate and unrealistic expectations of what will soon be available for relief and treatment of their loved ones, whom they would rather see not suffer. After all we have been told that if stem cells have this capacity to proliferate indefinitely and to differentiate into any type of tissue cell in the body, then if we could only learn how to control their intrinsic behaviour and function, we should be able to rebuild and restore whatever part of the body is malfunctioning or even missing.

That is a very lofty dream. **Nature seldom ever yields her deepest**

secrets easily and never does so completely. The path forward is always littered with multiple obstacles and challenges that must, of necessity, be painstakingly overcome. We may indeed make quantum leaps at times, but it is only through dogged determination and persistence in step-by-step, diligent and creative thinking and experimentation that slow and steady progress is made.

Yet, advances are being made in the stem cell arena almost every week. There are many bright minds and experienced clinicians working earnestly and consistently to master the many hurdles that must still be overcome before meaningful and practical clinical solutions can be found. That remains true even in the face of the amazing theoretical possibilities that stem cells can potentially deliver. Stem cell therapy with its prospects for restoring malfunctioning organs and tissues and even for rebuilding lost body parts, is indeed in sight, but practically speaking, even in the best doctor's offices and the most reputable hospitals everywhere, it remains a tantalizing silhouette on the research horizon. It is probably still fair to say that it is the realistic hope only for patients of future generations. When it comes to any kind of dramatic healing with stem cells, that sobering reality is worth repeating everywhere and all the time.

These possible dramatic advances are really in the field of Stem Cell Medicine. They relate almost exclusively to treating illness and disease. In that sense, they will become relevant after the fact – to patients who have suffered some acute event such as a heart attack or a spinal cord injury, or to those who experience chronic degenerative illness such as diabetes or Parkinson's disease, for example. On the other hand, Stem Cell Nutrition is all about the normal activity of repairing and maintaining the body before the clinical manifestations of any medical conditions. It is therefore fundamentally preventative in its application.

Nevertheless, it would be disappointing to complete a book in this area without at least reflecting on the significant progress that is being made in the area of stem cell- based therapy. For that reason, we have included a summary of some of the recent progress in this field in the **Appendix** at the back of the book.

12-Point
SUMMARY OF PART ONE

There is no doubt that we are on the cusp of a Stem Cell Revolution. This brief and inadequate review that was just presented will probably be somewhat out of date by the time you are reading this. Research in the field is moving fast. Nevertheless, some basic principles are clear. Let's enumerate them.

1. Pluripotent stem cells can proliferate and differentiate into almost every cell type in the human body.

2. Both embryonic stem cells and adult stem cells have shown the capacity to differentiate into the various cell types. Both types can now be cultured and conveniently manipulated.

3. Different tissue cell types (which all have the same DNA) can be induced by advanced biotechnology to regress and form new pluripotent stem cells that can differentiate thereafter into almost every other cell type.

4. When stem cells are injected into the blood stream or into local tissue sites that have been injured (or are malfunctioning), they are capable of proliferating and differentiating to repair (or replace) damaged cells in tissues or organs.

5. Stem cell release from the bone marrow can be stimulated to increase their number in circulation. This latter variable has been shown to affect the incidence, progression and prognosis for a number of common medical conditions.

6. Tissue repair or replacement with stem cells offers the interesting prospect of restoring function to damaged tissues and organs, seen in important degenerative and chronic illnesses.

7. Big challenges remain. Before any widespread application of stem cell therapy is realized, two big hurdles must be overcome: the tendency for rejection and the significant risk of inducing cancer.

8. Stem cell research around the world is intense and much progress is being made. There are many hopeful signs. It is certainly reasonable to anticipate that stem cell biotechnology will be on the forefront of medical advances in the years to come.

9. The natural spontaneous renewal system of the body has not received the same attention as the interventionist biotechnology that seeks to address disease states. That may be a big mistake.

10. The evidence to date points to this normal renewal system whereby stem cells routinely leave the bone marrow, circulate preferentially to injured tissue sites where they migrate to the specific locus of injury, then proliferate and differentiate into corresponding cells of the affected tissue.

11. The release of stem cells from the bone marrow is enhanced by factors also released by the injured tissue (G-CSF). Migration into the tissue is facilitated by cytokines (SDF-1), among other things.

12. The possibility of enhancing the normal renewal process – perhaps by a safer, more convenient and natural intervention - offers an alternate opportunity for exploiting the remarkable characteristics of stem cells to improve human health and well- being.

That final principle brings us to the interface with nutrition and the specific consideration of **Stem Cell Nutrition.** The practice of nutrition is as old as life itself, since all living things require input of raw materials. Throughout human history, dietary intake has been changing steadily – a process we choose to call 'The Evolution of Nutrition.' Just perhaps, the impact on stem cells may be the leading edge of this continuing evolution.

Could stem cells be affected in any significant way by something that we choose to eat, even as a dietary supplement? That's the subject of **Part Two** that follows immediately.

Part 1I

The Evolution of NUTRITION

evolution: *slow, gradual improvement; adapting to change or circumstance; spontaneous development*

Preamble to Part Two

If the new understanding of stem cells has triggered a possible *revolution* in medicine, then in contrast, the practice of nutrition has shown nothing but *evolution*, since it is as ancient as life itself. Just consider that the basic human consumption of plants and animals (including fish) has continued for many thousands of years as the natural means of sustenance and nourishment for maintaining life and health. In a word, we eat to live. Air, water and food are all truly indispensable ... the only real *sine qua non.*

Nutrition then is the cornerstone of life and the study of nutrition has become increasingly intense, especially over the last century when the appropriate tools became available. Today, books on nutrition could fill many a library. Authoritative and comprehensive textbooks in the field, like *Modern Nutrition in Health and Disease*, are too heavy to carry around. The subject is often linked to that of human metabolism and that field is even more vast in its scope. But despite the overwhelming complexity of the science, the basic information is too relevant to be ignored here.

The good news is that in this area, the academics and specialists do not have a monopoly on either information or experience. **Nutrition is every person's habit. The dietary traditions in every culture have been centuries in the making.** The best of nutritional practice has survived the test of time so that traditional experiences with consumption of foods and natural products justify their own existence by a fateful process of elimination. In normal daily living, people everywhere have discovered what's good for them and when bad choices have been made, the negative consequences taught the next generation what to avoid and how to take advantage of the good things nature has to offer.

In this preamble therefore, we want to take just a quick, cursory glance at this evolutionary process of nutrition. A sweeping panoramic tour through thousands of years of nutritional habit is designed therefore to give the reader a perspective only, not an education in the field. But it is an important perspective, so let's get to it.

FROM THE BEGINNING

Primitive man survived by simply hunting and gathering whatever was available and edible, until the so-called *Neolithic Revolution* – the first verifiable revolution in agriculture. During the Stone Age, widespread domestication of plants and animals over time, and in different parts of the known world, led to important social changes, including denser populations, more sedentary communities and early social stratification.

But nutrition hardly changed until much later when the so-called *British Agricultural Revolution* took place. Those changes were naturally made over a few centuries and so the terminology is somewhat questionable. If revolutions are by definition 'rapid', then this should hardly be designated as such. But at least it was 'accelerated' change, even if that was slow. Nevertheless, progressive legal protection of life, liberty and property encouraged personal initiative to build farms and to develop new farming tools and equipment.

Methods were invented for preservation and transportation of food and there was improvement in crop selection and farming methods. **The net result showed increases in productivity and the effective distribution of food.** This then reduced hunger and even famine during times of drought or crop disease. Similar developments were later seen on every continent.

Then came the *Industrial Revolution* of the 18th and 19th centuries with the introduction of machine-based manufacturing. There was the development of the steam engine leading to steam-powered railways and ships, and later the internal combustion engine and electrical power generation. What began in Great Britain, later spread to Europe, North America, Japan and eventually throughout the world. Industrialization led to urbanization and the new dense populations had to rely on the farmers in the old rural communities to supply the necessary food.

The truth is that despite thousands of years of human development leading up to the last century, nutrition had shown only slow gradual improvement, adapting to change and circumstance. It was indeed a process of natural, spontaneous development – so in a single word, there was only evolution. Food production was still done 'the old-fashioned way.' In three simple steps, it was grown, cooked and eaten. With urbanization, two more steps were added, so now it was grown, transported and sold - then cooked and eaten.

With further urbanization and industrialization in the 20th century, remarkable changes were made to growing and production, such as mechanical plowing, seeding and harvesting. Add fertilization and pesticides. Add changes to storage and preservation, with refrigeration and chemicals. Add electricity and efficient transportation. Add widespread refining methods – like the milling of grains to make flour or the polishing of rice with the removal of bran. Now we're into **the age of industrialized food**, especially since World War II. Food is now as much a product of technology as it is of agriculture.

WHATEVER BECAME OF FOOD?

Today the food industry has become the largest and most important in the world. Like all other industries, it is driven by forces of capitalism and profit, at least in the Western industrialized world. If market share and profit became the top priorities, nutrition is at best a secondary consideration. Were it not for the limited regulation by elected governments and the minimal but yet significant outcry of the public at times, who knows what modern nutrition would become in the fast-paced, media-manipulated, poorly-informed and confused, urban culture of the twenty first century?

However, it needs to be said that **food technology is not all about exploitation and abuse of consumers.** It is not all doom and gloom. Rather, there have been some outstanding achievements and benefits to the application of modern technology in the food industry. The sheer abundance of food at reasonable cost has gone a long way to eliminating large scale hunger, widespread malnutrition or even actual starvation. In fact, we hardly had a choice. Fifty years ago the world's population was only about half of what it is today. Only the massive increase in the use of hybrid seeds and chemical fertilizers allowed food production to be doubled to meet demand. Yet big challenges remain. We're running out of available land and the necessary water to meet the increasing need for an adequate food supply. But that's another matter.

Food is available today and adequate nutrition is almost universally possible, even in the most dense urban centers where the practice of agriculture is a forgotten and disregarded lifestyle. It is hard to imagine that only a century or two ago, large populations even in the developed world were subject to shortage and rationing of food. Yet in most communities, that remained a common occurrence.

There is such a wide variety of food available today, that it seems unreal that people suffered at different times, from diseases of nutrient deficiency. There were full-blown acute clinical illnesses like pellagra, scurvy or rickets. Although the underlying physiology was not understood for a long time, the widespread classic symptoms of deficiency were undeniably obvious. Today, these devastating conditions are relatively unknown, but although many still choose to deny it, there remains much evidence of chronic degenerative conditions that result from inadequate nutrient intake, but we'll have to come back to that.

Food technology not only increased the *quantity* of food available, but it also addressed another major problem. *Quality* control was also a significant issue especially with urbanization and increased population density. The decay and contamination of food sometimes led to food poisoning and other disease. But these problems were often either not apparent or generally ignored until the fateful consequences were observed. However, thanks to refrigeration, antioxidants, freeze-drying and other technology advances, food today is much better preserved and the incidence of *natural contamination* has ceased to be a really significant problem in industrialized nations.

Yet there is much more to the food story. ***Man-made contamination of food has become a real problem and that has had major health consequences.*** Today's food supply contains not inconsequential but deliberate additives for convenient processing, color, taste and preservation. Add to that, residual agricultural chemicals including hormones, antibiotics, pesticides and a host of other risky industrial and other pollutants. At the same time, commercial growing, handling, refining, storage and processing of foods does cause depletion of many essential nutrients so that even food by the same name, when compared to the equivalent product of an old-fashioned home garden, becomes a totally different nutritional product.

Two common examples should suffice. Think of planting some tomato seeds (which have not been genetically modified) at spring time in your own backyard vegetable garden. Then imagine picking a ripe appetizing tomato for your salad just before dinnertime in the summer. That's one thing. Now recall buying a "fresh" supermarket tomato which was picked green, sprayed with ethylene gas or with the chemical ethepan to ripen it, or buying it in a can with preservatives, or using it as ketchup (two thirds of which is sugar), or juice crystals (via vacuum puff-drying), or powder (via foam-mat drying). Yes, there is real natural tomato, and then there is everything else associated with tomato but is hardly that. Even if it goes by the same name, it cannot be the same thing.

For a second example, consider wheat. Whole wheat contains essential amino acids, fiber, vitamins and crucial minerals and trace elements. It is a very rich food. But then, leave it to the food processors to apply up to two dozen so-called refining steps, including high-pressure steel rolling, scouring, grinding and magnetic separation. All that refining is done to produce what exactly? A relatively tasteless, colorless, starchy material, with very low nutrient density, that we call 'white flour'. They remove the central wheat germ with so much nutritive goodness, and the high-fiber shell on the outside, with all those minerals. They discard the bulk of the nutrients in favor of the bland but stable residue. The end product may be cosmetically appealing perhaps and definitely more stable, but for nutritional purposes, it is essentially useless. And that's provided for human consumption. It is a cruel shame.

To add more insult to injury, **technology is now used not just to destroy good foods but to create synthetic foods.** Chemical technologists have now mastered the art of making food 'analogs', or imitation foods – all fabricated products. Because they are made by design, manufacturers can build-in whatever features they choose, to tantalize the ill-informed or careless consumer who could hardly distinguish 'fruit drinks' from 'fruit juices', or 'miracle whip' from real mayonnaise, or 'non-dairy creamer' from real milk, or 'textured protein' from real beef or bacon. The only limit to such nutritious sacrilege is the human imagination. It's all make-believe.

Then when you add the multi-billion dollar advertising campaigns, the subliminal entertainment and psychological abuse of children, the attractive packaging and universal exploitation of sensual taste buds – you've got a real epidemic in the making. It's the perfect nutritional storm, destroying the natural supply of essential nutrients in its wake. The ripple effects will be felt for generations to come.

THESIS -- ANTITHESIS

Someone else has pointed out that *'every thesis has its own antithesis, which in time gives rise to a new synthesis'*, (a philosophy attributed to Hegel). This classic dialectic is very true in the field of nutrition. With the increasing conversion from an essentially agricultural food supply to the ever popular industrialized food supply, the more informed interest groups have sought to emphasize, utilize and spread the word about the health dangers inherent in this shift. They have defended and fought for the preservation of an alternative food industry where the emphasis remains on nutritive value. They insist that feeding the body with the essentials it needs to maintain optimum health must remain the highest priority. They lobby everywhere against the use of pesticides and chemicals in farming, against the host of chemical additives in food; against deceptive labeling and packaging; against convenience and junk foods that especially appeal to children, and against much more. All this is done to preserve health and to promote wellness. That's a sacred value they choose to affirm and defend.

But let's not miss the critical point. The reality is that the human body has essential needs – it always has, it always will – long before changes in agriculture, industrialization, urbanization and modern technology. **The cell remains the same, its needs remain the same. The goal of good nutrition is to satisfy those unchanging needs.** When the food supply of the essential nutrients is inadequate or when food choices prove to be inappropriate (due to lifestyle, misinformation or advertising manipulation), then the reasonable alternative leads to food supplementation practices. And that's where we are today.

More and more, people of Western cultures have become aware and sensitive to the practical need for food supplements and ever since the second World War , there has been a succession of popular fads and trends that sought to capitalize on this new and increasing public awareness. That gave rise to a series of food supplement products that have addressed and emphasized different nutritional deficiencies and sometimes new health promotion opportunities. That's the subject of Chapter 4 that should take us to what was the leading edge in this field ... until recently.

QUID PRO QUO

Just before we get there, it may be useful to take a moment here to emphasize another critical point pertaining to nutrition and health. It is this: **every natural process in the human body seems to have a corresponding source in nature to supply the essential (or at least, the supportive) raw materials that address the potential need.** That would apply to the oxygen in the air we breathe and the water we have to drink. It could refer to the proteins that we eat to derive amino acids to maintain tissues and do the millions of other tasks both inside and outside the cells. It might be carbohydrates that supply energy or fiber that provide bulk for cleansing. Then there are vitamins to facilitate efficient metabolism and minerals for bone-strength, oxygen transport and much more. We could also mention antioxidants for cellular protection, and fatty acids for specialized roles in cell membranes, and so on.

You get the point. **Nature's food provides externally, what nature's cells need internally.** It's a kind of natural *quid pro quo.* So, long before our understanding of biology, and long before the focus on nutrition, there has always been this intrinsic supply from nature. There has been this provision of a wide variety of nutrients, as well as what are now referred to as 'nutraceuticals.' This latter term refers to *foods or food products* that can, in principle, provide health and medical benefits. Since the more common term, 'pharmaceuticals', refers only to *drugs* designed and manufactured with such benefits in mind, the new term offers hope of some similar clinical effects but with the emphasis on the natural, nutritious source that food really is.

Now then, since nutrients and nutraceuticals support intrinsic physiological processes and needs in the human body, it might very well be expected that for any natural renewal system in the body, such as we saw in Part One, there would exist some foods, or nutrients in foods, that might enhance (or at least support) this universal renewal system. And there is. This is what **Stem Cell Nutrition** implies and that is why it is now **the leading edge of nutrition in the 21st century.**

In the next chapter we'll review the basics of **'Supplementation 101'** and highlight the various approaches to enhance dietary intake in pursuit of optimal health and wellness. We'll recount the story of how we got to the new leading edge of nutritional supplementation in Chapter 5 and then provide some details of its application in Chapter 6. The story now becomes even more interesting ...

CHAPTER 4

Supplementation 101:
A Review

Food technology made a major leap forward in the West after the end of World War II. All aspects of the food industry from production to consumption were definitely affected. Let's just follow that sequence, shall we.

THE FOOD CHAIN

The food chain begins with the soil. This is the normal source of trace elements but these become depleted with successive crops, so technology has employed the benefits of chemistry to add commercial fertilizers. These fertilizers however, provide mainly nitrogen to increase crop yields, not the deficient minerals to improve health. Some fertilizers even deplete essential nutrients like iron, vitamin C and an essential amino acid (lycine), with more negative consequences up the food chain[1]. Livestock fare little better. They are routinely fed more supplements than humans, but they also get the undesirable antibiotics, hormones and hormone-like substances to maximize their yield in terms of profit margin. Again, these practices have potentially long-term risks, if not hazards to human health[2].

Harvesting also plays a role in nutrition. Typically, commercial fruits and vegetables are picked and gathered while not yet ripe, to satisfy demands for transportation and marketing. The reality is that the nutrient content is only fully realized when the product is ripened in situ. Vitamin C levels, for example, could be as low as 25-35% for green produce picked mechanically, when compared to a vine ripened alternative[1].

Then the typical raw food has to be handled, transported and stored. These all reduce nutrient content, whether by convenient slicing and cutting, canning, necessary warehousing and shelf storage, inescapable light exposure, inevitable enzyme degradation, and more.

Then comes the big one: food processing. This activity causes the major loss of nutrients from foods in industrialized society. That's what we do ourselves, in the home. We peel fruit, cook (boil) vegetables, slice onions, toast bread, can peaches, stir-fry raw foods, barbecue meats, and the list goes on. Add to that, what the industry does. Consider all the highly processed, convenience and junk foods. These are products for consumers' pleasure and manufacturers' profits. But they do little good and often a lot of harm to the human body.

It's not all bad though. Some processing can destroy harmful pathogens or partially release nutrients to increase bioavailability (when done only in moderation, obviously). Food processing and preparation can also improve appearance, taste and texture, which could all enhance appeal and intake to arguably favor nutrition, if and when foods are appropriately chosen. But overprocessing rules the day. **Many studies have confirmed the deleterious effects that extreme processing has on the nutritional value of foods**[1,3]. Some nutrient losses are just moderate, but some are severe enough to cause genuine alarm. So-called 'junk food' is not worthy of any further comment. The name says it all.

Attempts to restore nutritive value to foods by putting back (with chemical additives) what was removed or lost in process, has proved to be woefully inadequate. It may be a trick of the trade, proven to be effective with some consumers. But living cells cannot be fooled by any form of advertising and promotions. They only recognize the real thing, and that is and always will be the only real thing: valuable nutrients that practically enter the actual cells of the body.

If the industrialization of food that was just discussed above represents the 'thesis' we mentioned earlier, what's the 'antithesis'? In the latter part of the 20th century, **a spontaneous movement took hold**. It could hardly be called a movement since it had neither organization nor leadership. It was instead driven by a philosophy of wholesome food and responsible nutrition, leading subsequently to better health and wellness. Enlightened consumers and health advocates became alarmed by the depletion of nutrients in highly processed, convenience and junk foods. They also warned against the potential toxicity of the commercial food chain, with all the chemical additives and physical manipulation of raw foods. They popularized a new profitable health food industry that provided 'natural' and 'organic' foods as the alternative. They were anxious to choose organic foods (grown in soils organically prepared, with no chemical pesticides and no synthetic substances added before or after harvesting). They were willing to pay the price for more natural products. They wanted raw, unprocessed food that was hopefully fresh and devoid of all the additives otherwise added for taste, color, stability, processing and so on.

Such organic and natural foods were obviously an insurmountable challenge for large commercial food companies. Their products were driven by market necessities and were therefore limited by existing technologies, if worldwide demand was ever to be met. However, the demand/supply forces have allowed the availability of more natural wholesome foods to increase over decades and today that represents a truly viable alternative lifestyle choice in most western societies. Since, as Adele Davis pointed out decades ago, 'you are what you eat', then **it is incumbent on the responsible individual to choose foods wisely and carefully.**

To that end, here is an unauthorized, but clearly unassailable list of personal nutrition guidelines:

Ten Recommendations for Good Nutrition

1. Eat Small, Regular and Varied Meals.   (Choose rainbow colors.)
2. Drink at least 8 Glasses of Fluid daily.   (Water, juices, milk?)
3. Favor foods with a low Glycemic Index.(Cut back refined sugars.)
4. Run away from Fat.   (Keep essential fatty acids.)
5. Eat as many Raw Foods as possible.   (Increase fiber.)
6. Shop for Health.   (Read labels carefully.)
7. Avoid Crash Diets.   (They will make you crash!)
8. Practice only responsible fasting.   (Make it short, break it slowly.)
9. Treat yourself occasionally.   (Nutrition is fun too!)
10. Supplement Your Diet

That list of suggestions is included here primarily to emphasize the last one. It is by no means the least. About every four years, the US Food and Drug Administration (USFDA) issues new dietary guidelines for consumers. Those consist essentially of a Food Pyramid designed to help people make healthy food choices. Their impact in real terms is truly limited but they have the unintended consequence perhaps of supporting the US industrial food establishment. The Food Pyramid provides at best, a false sense of security, for it fails to address real practical nutritional values, even in the best of normal supermarket foods.

Clinical nutrition is a specialized practice in the care and management of patients with diagnosed illness. Supplementation however, is a wise lifestyle alternative even for healthy individuals, to provide a guaranteed supply of essential nutrients to the body, on a regular basis and in a convenient form. It is in essence, first and foremost, a form of **nutritional insurance.** We live in an age of busy lifestyles, an industrialized food supply, commonly poor food choices, and excessive demands from the stress and pollutants in our environment. It has become very difficult in contemporary society to find the ingredients for a truly healthy diet and to make consumption of the same a regular lifestyle pattern. Under such circumstances, you can ensure that you get what your cells need by the careful and responsible use of food supplements that provide all the basic essentials.

WHY SUPPLEMENTS?

The Food and Drug Administration (FDA) regulates dietary supplements as a category of foods, and not as drugs. They therefore do not require FDA approval prior to entry into the consumer marketplace. At the same time however, no legal claims can be made for such dietary supplements to cure, mitigate or treat any specific disease or medical condition. Yet companies that market dietary supplements are permitted to make structure/function claims about a given supplement in their marketing materials, but only after adequate substantiation and FDA notification.

In 2009, the FDA finally announced a rule establishing regulations to require current good manufacturing practices (GMP) for all dietary supplements, but enforcement is difficult and costly, so quality assurance remains a major challenge in this industry.

There has been much controversy and debate for decades, in both North America and Europe regarding the need for dietary supplementation and the safety of this lifestyle practice. While that debate continues, **more and more people are discovering that simple nutritional intervention and lifestyle changes are making signif-icant positive impact on the quality of their lives** in general, and their health status in particular. A study sponsored by the Centers for Disease Control and Prevention's National Center for Health Statistics, found that more than 40 percent of Americans used sup-plements from 1988 to 1994, and more than half took vitamins from 2003 to 2006[4]. Multivitamins were found to be the most common-ly used supplement. These more aware consumers relate in some way to a cause that is being championed by the so-called 'health freedom movement'. But that is only a loose coalition of comple-mentary medicine organizations, practitioners, consumers, activists and producers of natural products. They want increased availability and less government regulation of complementary/alternative thera-pies, in general, and of nutritional supplements in particular.

Let's also observe that the **overwhelming majority of people who use dietary supplements on a regular basis tend to be the most nutritionally informed consumers among the general public**. They are the same people who read food labels carefully. They also make deliberate lifestyle choices that more often than not promote better health and wellbeing. They eat less junk food, exercise more, share environmental concerns, smoke less, are more weight con-scious and tend to avoid abuse of alcohol and drugs. They deserve more praise and recognition for their exemplary habits in a culture that seems generally to be moving in the opposite direction in many of these same areas.

Nutritional supplementation by the general public ought never to be confused with medical treatment. Their roles are completely differ-ent. We will come back to this much later in this book, but suffice it to point out here, that the focus of supplementation must always be on the prevention of illness and the promotion of better health and wellbeing. The vast majority of dietary supplements are daily consumed by fairly normal, otherwise healthy individuals who wish to enjoy a benefit today rather than risk some avoidable disaster tomorrow. Better health and quality of life is the ultimate goal.

Orthodoxy suggests that the promotion of adequate and balanced dieting is the way to go. The dietary establishment insists that you'll get it all if you eat right. But the results show that despite the abundance of food available, the typical North American diet leaves much to be desired. We eat meals high in sugar and empty calories, laden with fat, salt and food additives, and low in vegetables, fruits and fibre. Despite our best limited efforts to date, the tide has not turned in the general public. Therefore, **supplementation remains for many people the most practical alternative to guarantee the regular intake of essential nutrients.**

That leads us to consider another critical question: What foods or nutrients are truly essential? As more nutritional information has come to light and as more research has been done on the content and value of many ancient and traditional foods, herbs and other natural products, there has been an expanding range of important food derivatives in the public/media spotlight. Starting after the last World War when the application of technology was widely expanded, increasing public awareness of nutrient deficiencies and subsequent market availability led to progressive trends in the focus of the food supplement industry. It seemed like every decade, there would be some new 'breakthrough' in understanding human physiology and therefore impacted the relevance of some new 'type of supplement' to meet some identifiable but previously overlooked need of the human body in search of optimum health and wellness.

We will review these trends in turn, starting with vitamin supplements in the nineteen fifties and leading up to where we are today, at the leading edge defined by the discovery of the body's natural renewal system. Recall that stem cells leave the bone marrow and migrate to tissues in need of repair or replacement, all the time. We cannot emphasize enough that **everybody has stem cells; everybody uses stem cells; everybody uses stem cells every day; stem cells work ... and they work every time.** Could Stem Cell Nutrition be a key to enhance that natural renewal process? ... That's the leading edge of nutrition today, as we shall see (or even better, as we shall prove).

But we dare not get ahead of ourselves. So we go back to the fifties, when vitamin supplements were just coming to the marketplace in force. That trend introduced a whole new world of nutritional ideas to concerned consumers.

VITAMINS

In this whirl-wind supplementation tour, we begin with Vitamins because this was the first class of nutrients known to be essential to life and at the same time, suspected for deficiency in the diet. Clearly there are extreme vitamin deficiency diseases like pellagra (due to deficiency of vitamin B6 or niacin), or scurvy (vitamin C deficiency), or beri-beri (vitamin B1 or thiamine deficiency) and night-blindness (vitamin A deficiency). Those extreme conditions were, for obvious reasons, quite prevalent in certain populations many decades ago. Although they have not been totally eradicated, what is even more common today is that which is referred to as 'sub-clinical deficiency'. But what does that mean?

Most doctors would insist that malnutrition is rare in affluent Western societies. They assume that with such an abundant food supply and in the absence of some deficiency diagnosis, patients are clinically okay and there's nothing more to be concerned about except perhaps weight management and encouraging 'good eating habits'. That's usually the common response in the typical doctor's office whenever patients make comments or ask questions about nutrition in general.

But on this issue, maybe the doctor is not the best person to consult, because invariably, their medical training significantly influences their diagnostic paradigm. **In the area of contemporary nutrition, many doctors are often ill-informed, with very little interest in such matters.** Only slowly is the more recent nutritional information filtering into their office (and often from educated patients, by the way). In fairness to doctors and other healthcare personnel however, their respective professional boards or colleges do hold sway on how and what they are at liberty to recommend to patients. So if they 'err' on the side of caution it may be quite understandable.

There is no need to present a persuasive case for vitamin supplementation in this brief review. Some groups are clearly more at risk than others. These include women of all ages, the aged, low income groups (that tend to eat poor diets), people with chronic disease, the immuno-compromised, patients with prolonged drug use, smokers and others. But if any reader needs to find a reason for taking vitamin supplements in general, consider this. Vitamins are indispensable to human life. They play vital roles in healthy metabolism. Yet the human body cannot make them, they must be ingested. In principle, they can all be obtained from a truly adequate and balanced diet. But knowing what we all know about the nutrient quality of the food supply and the nature of dietary intake across the board, the wisest response must surely be to opt for **nutritional insurance.**

After all, what's to oppose a considered lifestyle choice that assures a guaranteed supply of essential nutrients on a regular basis in a convenient form? Any sensible and concerned person should at least do a risk-benefit analysis before coming to any conclusion. The potential benefit is certainly on the table at least and the risk is minimal in normal dosages. (High dose megavitamin therapy proposed by practitioners of Orthomolecular Medicine is a different matter and should only be considered, at least under expert professional care). When it comes to essential nutrients, the simple rationale here is no less than the old adage, 'better safe than sorry.' Let's illustrate.

Just imagine that for years, some unfortunate mothers had given birth to babies with neural tube defects. Finally, after much careful research it was finally concluded that the malformation was associated with previously unknown folic acid deficiency in expectant mothers[5]. This led to government regulations insisting on folate supplementation for women of child-bearing age[6]. That's just one example of the intrinsic benefit from sensible nutritional insurance derived from simply making good quality vitamin intake and other forms of nutrient supplementation a regular lifestyle habit. It's a healthy choice worth making that supersedes any residual risk that you might be afraid of taking.

And what risk is there of taking vitamin supplements in normal amounts on a daily basis? Just note that the water-soluble vitamins (Vitamin C and the eight essential B's) are regularly secreted from the body when necessary. Although the fat-soluble vitamins (A, D, E and K) can theoretically accumulate in the fatty tissues, that observation is practically rare in normal use and even so, is readily reversible on discontinued use. Vitamin D in particular has now come into focus and many doctors are regularly encouraging their patients to use supplementary intake to avoid symptoms of deficiency, which the evidence suggests have become more clinically relevant across the board in North America[7-9]. This is particularly relevant to breastfed infants, older adults and people with dark skin, limited sun exposure or reduced fat absorption. Again, that medical interest was all *after the fact*.

Of course, as we learned more about vitamins and vitamin-deficiency, we also devised how to synthesize and manipulate many of them in the laboratory. But when it comes to food, it is difficult to duplicate nature. **Natural food is packaged as whole foods** - not isolated ingredients. The package is designed by nature for maximum bioavailability and efficacy. Therefore, it is always preferable to utilize 'natural source' vitamins – packed with all the important co-factors and support players – rather than synthetic alternatives. For example, rose hips, acerola cherries or fresh lemons will deliver precious bioflavonoids that just don't accompany 'synthetic' ascorbic acid. They therefore provide a better source of Vitamin C.

Since the 1950's the healthy lifestyle habit of taking supplementary vitamins has become a 'given' among the so-called 'health and wellness community.' These are the people who since that time, continue to educate themselves about food, nutrition, lifestyle and more. They choose to take responsibility for themselves, for their diet, for their health and for their future. So should you.

ESSENTIAL FATTY ACIDS

Ever since the first vitamins were discovered at the beginning of the last century, it was suspected that there would be more essential dietary ingredients to be identified. Not all would turn out to be vital – *amines* as Casimir Funk conjectured. In fact, most vitamins do not conform to his description of 'organic compounds that contain nitrogen.' Nonetheless, when the two essential fatty acids (EFA's), alpha-linoleic acid (omega-3) and linolenic acid (omega-6) were first discovered in 1923 they were designated the label 'vitamin F'. But by 1930, it was clear that they were better classified with the fats than with the known vitamins. They were not amines alright, but they were still vital. They were 'essential' because the human body requires them for good health but cannot synthesize them endogenously. They must be obtained from dietary sources.

The most common food sources for essential fatty acids are fish (especially fatty deep water fish like salmon, mackerel and sardines) and shell fish, as well as some vegetable oils (compressed), flaxseed, sunflower and pumpkin seeds, leafy vegetables and walnuts.

The two essential fatty acids are chemically short-chain, polyunsaturated fatty acids which the body uses to make other longer chain and more desaturated fatty acids such as EPA, DHA, GLA and AA which all have long names that would only distract us here. But more importantly, those latter fatty acids serve many different biological functions, especially with regard to the immune response and inflammation (the body's natural and universal response to all types of insult or injury). EFA's are also believed to play an important role in the regulation of cholesterol, the lowering of blood pressure and the maintenance of cardiac rhythm[10,11]. Research has shown that higher intakes of fish and omega-3 fatty acids are somewhat effective in the treatment of minor depression. It could also be linked to decreased rates of major depression[12]. Clinically, however, extreme EFA deficiency manifests principally in dermatitis (skin disorder).

What's the lesson to be gained here? **Nutrition must always be balanced.** It is tempting at times to eliminate one or more component from the diet but there are always unintended consequences. Consider this. As a class of foods, 'Fat' has got a bad name, especially at a time when obesity and its consequences have become an epidemic in society, at all ages. That's even true despite the media obsession with leanness. So, the temptation might be to avoid all fat. That would be wrong. Fat is basically a good thing for the body, providing essential nutrients like the omega-3 and omega-6 fatty acids we discuss here, as well as being an important source of physical energy and body warmth. We need fats and oils in the diet providing lipids in the body for cell membranes, body structure, healthy skin, reproduction, hormones and bile, essential nutrients, warmth and protection. Therefore, let's keep the balance. While trying to reduce the excessive levels of fat consumption, let's also be careful to maintain adequate intake of essential fatty acids, in particular.

HERBALS

The National Center for Complementary and Alternative Medicine released a survey in 2004 showing that among US adults age 18 and over, herbal therapy was a commonly used alternative therapy, second only to vitamins and minerals[13]. A good case could be made for the widespread use of particular herbs as dietary supplements but any attempts to use them in a truly therapeutic sense to treat or cure disease, except in the case of real professionals, is at best unwarranted and foolhardy, at least in the modern industrialized world. At worst, it could even be dangerous[14].

Yet it should be pointed out that even today, half the world's population still uses herbs on a regular basis as their primary source of medicinal remedies[15]. This could also be justified in the absence of other proven therapeutics and in cultures with historic traditions and well-established (though old-fashioned) remedies and protocols, at much less cost.

Even in our society, where there are common chronic complaints, there is certainly a place for safe, natural alternative interventions such as herbal supplementation to help relieve the common symptomatology. There is no doubt that many herbs provided by nature contain ingredients that have important therapeutic value to the human body. Herbs can provide several phytochemical precursors for body functions. These natural products then help the body to perform important metabolic processes that add up to better overall health. Herbs also tend to be a good source of natural antioxidants which are vital protectors of cells from the toxic free radicals that are now implicated in the pathogenesis of many disease conditions.

Any given herbal supplement product may contain all the compounds naturally found in a plant, or it may have just one or two of the chemicals that have been successfully isolated. The quality can vary quite significantly. It may be blended with other ingredients for any number of reasons and one should always be cautious in the selection of such products. To make sensible choices one should first be reliably informed of known benefits to be derived, at least by tradition. The typical herb goes back hundreds, if not thousands of years. Cumulative experience should then define its value. Any known adverse effects should be noted. Reports of any clinical trials would be more than helpful. And finally, the source is vitally important. One should insist on reputable manufacturers/suppliers and take time to read labels which should be self-explanatory and fairly complete. The claim that something is 'standardized', 'certified' or 'verified' provides no guarantee of a higher quality product, since these terms are all legally unspecified and unregulated. Therefore, *caveat emptor* (buyer beware!).

Many herbal supplements can act in the same way as drugs, at least in the broadest of terms. This should not be surprising since **many drugs on the market today are derived from natural herbs which first attracted research because of their reputation for therapeutic effects**[16]. But herbs themselves act without the specificity and controlled distribution of researched pharmaceutical preparations. They can cause medical problems if not used correctly, or if taken in excessive amounts. More often than not though, in normal use, any side effects from herbal supplements will tend to be mild, self-limiting and usually readily reversible. Pregnant women, nursing mothers and small children would be wise to avoid unnecessary use of herbal products, just to err on the safe side.

There is a wide variety of herbs in use in North America today. Some are commonly available in supermarkets, health food stores or at the Alternative Medicine sections of some pharmacies. Others find more limited use by complementary healthcare professionals like naturopaths, herbalists and chiropractors. And that's probably how it should be.

When considering herbs and herbal products, the issue is clearly not related to supplementing the body's need for essential nutrients. That has always been and probably will always remain the proper and traditional function of normal food. But what nature needs, nature always provides. It is therefore quite appropriate to broaden that rather narrow understanding of 'essential nutrients' and gain appreciation for the consumption of natural products for other reasons. If 'essential' means 'necessary for life and *avoiding death*', then obviously the so-called essential nutrients remain the only focus. But if we broaden the use of the key word 'essential' to mean 'beneficial for life and *promoting health*', then that invites us to explore more of what we already know. We do know that **some plant products available in nature, although not formally regarded as foods, seem designed to provide the body with benefits that improve the quality of life and health and may even as a consequence, prolong life.** It is in that healthful context that we shall come to Stem Cell Nutrition. But we must be patient in getting there.

FIBER

Edible or dietary fiber is a remarkable component of food. For a very long time it was regarded as the residual waste left behind after all the useful nutrients had been digested and absorbed from the gastrointestinal tract. It was more like a non-food than an actual nutrient. And yet it turns out that the very properties of indigestibility and non-absorption make fiber an indispensable ingredient in normal food intake. It is indeed an essential nutrient that exerts a number of beneficial effects both on the walls and muscular action of the intestines and on the digesting contents as they make their way through the body after being consumed.

The plant polysaccharides and lignins which are resistant to hydrolysis by the human digestive enzymes fall into two broad categories. Soluble fiber (gums, mucillages, pectins) is readily fermented in the colon into gases and physiologically active by- products. Insoluble fiber (cellulose, lignin, hemicelluloses) essentially absorbs water and provides bulking but it can sometimes be partially fermented in the colon too.

Today, it is clear that dietary fiber has at least three important effects on the digestive contents. First, it increases motility, thereby reducing transit time. Secondly, fiber helps to bind and absorb many potentially harmful substances and prevents them from building up and becoming a toxic load in the body. Thirdly, fiber can apparently modify several significant compounds before absorption, including bile salts, cholesterol and triglycerides. These are all healthy consequences from adequate fiber intake.

Some disadvantages do exist with high fiber in the diet. There is the potential for significant intestinal gas production and subsequent bloating. Plus, if insufficient fluid is consumed, constipation can occur.

On average, North Americans eat so much highly processed, refined, convenience and junk foods, that daily consumption of fiber is far too low. This correlates with the increased intake of empty calories and contributes to the recent epidemic of obesity and all those negative clinical, economic and social consequences. The situation has become so bad, that the US FDA has given approvals for food product manufacturers to make health claims for fiber[17]. **Diets rich in fiber are to be promoted for all normal individuals.**

One further observation should be made before leaving this subject of dietary fiber. It's namely this: Again, we are witnessing nature at work with unprogrammed (no human intervention) efficiency. Long before humans understood the varied physiological benefits to be derived from high fiber intake, those who consumed it were deriving all the same advantages that we have recently come to appreciate. In other words, the value of nutrition is to be emphasized as an intrinsic value, whereby all the ingredients of good, safe, natural food, perform all their physiological function without any conscious direction, without specification and without any imposed limitation. **Natural sources provide ingredients that are spontaneous solutions to the body's needs.** They are designed for real effectiveness, destined to produce better health and well-being and in the famous words of NASA, ' they deliver'! Stem cells will demonstrate that same quality from nature as we shall see when Stem Cell Nutrition comes under the spotlight later. That's something to anticipate.

ANTIOXIDANTS

Human life can be sustained for months without food and days without water, but it only takes minutes without oxygen for cells to begin dying off. Indeed, oxidation reactions are crucial for life. All cellular metabolic activity begins there. Oxidation produces energy - and no energy, no life. Nothing is more vital.

However, there is a paradox of metabolism. Oxidation reactions can produce some lethal intermediates called free radicals. These highly reactive species are toxic to cells. They initiate chain reactions in cells and on cell membranes that left unchecked would be lethal, causing damage or death to cells. Therefore, they must be stopped. That's where antioxidants come in. These are molecules that inhibit these chain reactions by quenching the reactive oxygen species (ROS) or free radical intermediates. They do this by being oxidized themselves – like molecular sacrificed lambs. But that's not the whole story. They are not suicidal. They only act the part. They have the ability to cycle in repeated reduction – oxidation so they are not generally consumed as they do their job. The antioxidants give up hydrogen or electrons to the free radicals and other ROS and then take them back elsewhere.

The ROS produced in cells include hydrogen peroxide, hypochlorous acid and free radicals such as the hydroxyl radical and the superoxide anion. Of these, the hydroxyl radical is particularly unstable and tends to react most indiscriminately with almost all biological molecules. When any ROS attacks DNA for example, mutations obviously can occur that if left unchecked, can cause cancer. When they attack lipids in cell membranes, cellular integrity is compromised and that can lead to cell death.

It's no wonder that cells have intrinsic mechanisms to oppose this destructive premature oxidation. These are natural free radical scavengers that do the important but dirty work. There are important enzymes that are exceedingly efficient at this – namely, superoxide dismutase, methionine reductase, catalase and glutathione peroxidase. The cells make these enzymes for their own defence as a normal matter of course. And in addition, their continuous work is daily supplemented by nutritional intake of other molecular antioxidants that include vitamins A, C and E (they ACE! this assignment every time), the supportive minerals selenium and zinc, and other nutrients. Also, it should be mentioned that some important metabolic intermediates (products of other cellular reactions) are functional antioxidants. These include glutathione, lipoic acid, uric acid and ubiquinol (coenzyme Q10).

Without a doubt, the relative importance and interactions between such a variety of antioxidants becomes very complicated. Suffice it to say that they all work together synergistically to perform the important job of defending cell integrity and metabolism. Each antioxidant has its own role to perform and does it when it's available and called upon.

That brings us to the question of antioxidant availability. Dietary intervention cannot change everything pertaining to premature oxidation and cell death, but it can change a lot. Ever since it was discovered that vitamins A, C, and E were effective antioxidants – that spawned a revolution: the antioxidant revolution[18]. We could affect the availability of these ACE vitamins by dietary intake. There was a critical handle on the problem of oxidative stress which can be a killer. That meant increasing the consumption of fresh fruits and vegetables – making the best dietary meals look like a rainbow. As if we did not already have enough reason, now everyone must be encouraged to eat like that. Eat your spinach and broccoli, go after those citrus fruits and don't forget the edible nuts and seeds. That's A, C and E for you.

Then again, there is always the opportunity for guaranteed nutritional insurance with supplements where indicated. It has also meant looking for other antioxidant supplements to complete a symphony of defensive players. So here they come. Glutathione precursors are first on deck.

Glutathione precursors
The cell's major internal antioxidant is a tripeptide molecule called glutathione. It has been sometimes designated as the 'master antioxidant' in the hierarchy. This critical cell-protector is only synthesized inside cells and from three amino acids: cysteine (with an 'e'), glutamic acid and glycine. Of these, cysteine is the rate-limiting component. It is an essential amino acid only obtained from the diet. However, most importantly, it gets across the cell membrane only in dimeric form, as cystine (without the 'e'), which is found principally in undenatured bovine whey proteins and in the proteins found in Mother's breast milk[19]. The challenge is to get adequate amounts of dietary cysteine, for which carefully prepared whey protein concentrate is a convenient supplementary source.

Glutathione has labile sulfhydryl (or thiol) groups, designated as -SH (hence the label, GSH), which is the basis of its powerful antioxidant action in cells. The hydrogen atom attached to the sulphur undergoes reversible transfer which gives GSH this strong affinity for oxygenated (or oxidized) species. This is the basis of the cell's principal internal defence against premature oxidation and insults from free radicals, some infectious agents and potential carcinogens. Glutathione is well known for its ability to enhance the immune system, to neutralize free radicals, to regulate other antioxidants in the cell and to help detoxify both exogenous chemicals and endogenous metabolites[20].

Many attempts have been made to enhance glutathione but beside the use of whey protein concentrate,[20,21] other approaches have proved ineffective for any sustained benefit. GSH itself is easily digested in the intestines but when injected, it has a short half life in the circulation. Chemically altered GSH tends to be metabolized to harmful or even toxic products, such as alcohol and acetaldehyde. As a lone amino acid, cysteine tends to be associated with toxicity and is itself readily metabolized. The drug n-acetyl cysteine (NAC) has been used intravenously as an acute treatment for Tylenol overdose. Orally, its bioavailability is about 10% and its effect on glutathione levels is only temporary. Another drug labelled OTZ is also a cysteine precursor but is subject to feedback inhibition.

In the final analysis, therefore, cysteine dipeptides (cystine) are available in the diet. When carefully prepared as convenient whey protein concentrates and used as a dietary supplement, published results demonstrate an increase of up to 30% in the glutathione levels of normal individuals[22]. Since the intracellular synthesis of glutathione is subject to feedback regulation, it is reasonable to conclude that even in normal individuals, there is health benefit to be derived from such lifestyle practice.

We emphasize once again that since natural cell protection requires adequate GSH synthesis and because this synthesis is limited by the availability of cysteine precursors in the diet, nature does provide its own sources as the solution. That's the basic observation or principle at work. **Natural cellular defence requires it, so natural food sources provide it.** In the same way, if the natural renewal system of the body requires the release of stem cells from the bone marrow (as it does!), it should not surprise us to find a natural food source to enhance the release and migration of those very stem cells to maintain and restore normal tissues, everywhere and all the time. That's the point to be made here. It's important, as the stage is being set.

Phytonutrients

Phytochemicals are nothing more than chemicals manufactured by plants. They are all natural and many have biological significance, especially as antioxidants. It is now generally accepted that many of the health benefits attributed to high intake of brightly coloured fruits and vegetables, as well as many nuts and edible seeds, can be reasonably attributed to the phytochemicals – more precisely, phytonutrients – that they contain. Hundreds of these have been identified and many of them are being actively studied around the world. We'll arbitrarily pick out perhaps the leading antioxidant in this class and give just a short focused review.

That focus is on *resveratrol*, a polyphenol that the media picked up on to help account for what is known as the "French Paradox". This refers to the fact that although the French consume a diet relatively rich in saturated fat, they suffer an unexpected low incidence of coronary heart disease. The popular TV program *CBS 60 Minutes* aired a description of this paradox in the US in 1991 and included the proposal that red wine, or alcohol, decreases the incidence of cardiac diseases. The theory was that one or more of the ingredients in red wine (which to the French is somewhat like 'water to fish') potentially helped the heart. Early signs pointed to resveratrol. That turned on the spotlight worldwide to red wine as a possible protection for the heart and increased the sale and consumption of red wine noticeably. But like so much else in the media, that was a rush to judgment. Research is continuing, but the evidence shows very low concentrations of resveratrol in red wine. The active ingredients to possibly account for the paradox seem more likely to be *oligomeric proanthrocyanidins (OPCs)* [23].

Be that as it may, resveratrol remains a very important and bioactive phytochemical. It is associated with a number of potential health benefits, such as anti-cancer, anti-viral, neuroprotective, anti-aging and anti-inflammatory effects, all of which have been demonstrated *in vitro* and reported[24]. Clinical trials of resveratrol are continuing.

Resveratrol is produced naturally by several plants and in particular, it is found in the seeds, skins and pulp (usually in that declining order) of different grapes (for example, muscadine) and berries (like acai or goji). Nutritional supplements made from these sources have gained widespread acceptance and more recently, the dried root of a Japanese knotweed has been used as an alternate economical, concentrated source.

DIGESTIVE ENZYMES

Enzymes are biological catalysts. They can be divided into three broad categories: (i) Food enzymes that are present in raw foods and start the digestive process; (ii) digestive enzymes that convert large complex food molecules into smaller absorbable units, and (iii) metabolic enzymes which maintain living cells and essentially run our bodies.

The key point here is that the normal processing of foods, whether by the food industry or in the home kitchen, destroys food enzymes. The food that may look and even taste the same, could be as different from the real thing as chalk is from cheese. One with no enzymes (and therefore no life), is to be contrasted with the live, enzyme-rich composition of healthy food as found in nature. Only raw food is certain to deliver the latter. Those food enzymes were designed in nature to initiate the digestive process and when absent, there is an additional burden on the human digestive system. That system is therefore, at times overwhelmed, and food passes through the entire gut undigested, with incomplete absorption.

The simple observation is that nutrition ultimately is designed to feed cells. The 7-step process begins with ingestion, but that must be followed then by digestion, absorption, circulation, migration into cells, intracellular metabolism and finally, elimination of residual and metabolic waste. That chain is no stronger than its weakest link.

All uncooked foods contain an abundance of food enzymes which correspond to the type of nutrients they provide. Those foods with relatively high fat content like dairy and edible oils, contain higher concentrations of the fat digesting enzyme, lipase. Grains which provide carbohydrates also contain higher concentrations of amylase and less lipase or proteases. Lean meats, on the other hand, are a good source of protein and they contain protease in the form of cathepsin and little amylase. Even low caloric foods like fruits and vegetables have mainly the important cellulose enzymes to help break down the plant fibers. All these food enzymes spare the body the extra digestive burden. That's why plants grown on healthy, mineral-rich soils, absorb the elements they require to make generous amounts of enzymes. This they do in spades, especially during the ripening process.

There is no substitute for food enzymes. There is only one enzyme factory on the face of the earth and that is the living cell. Only nature knows how to manufacture food enzymes. No chemist or drug company or laboratory can. Therefore we must harvest and consume nature's product. Antacids, synthetic digestive aids and motility agents are not enzymes and they are no substitutes for them either.

There is a limited enzyme potential in the body. When food enzymes do some of the digestive work, less demand is made on the digestive enzymes in the body and more of that potential is then reserved for the all important metabolic enzymes that maintain health. But many people face a kind of enzyme depletion and sometimes bankruptcy, when they attempt to survive on food devoid of its natural enzymes. The practice of dietary supplementation with live enzymes (derived exclusively from raw plant foods) would certainly be another wise contemporary lifestyle choice.

Improving digestion can only help to facilitate the nutrients that we consume in getting to their ultimate destination – inside cells. That brings us to our last category of nutritional supplementation as we wrap up our whirlwind tour. It's all preparatory to the excitement of arriving at the leading edge in the next chapter. We conclude here with the mention of a nutrient delivery system – a kind of biological FedEx or UPS. Now, how about that?

NUTRIENT DELIVERY SYSTEMS

Some scientists involved in the area of food supplementation have addressed the delivery process to investigate methods that could, in principle, enhance the nutrient delivery system. Perhaps the most promising approach was the one first developed by the late Dr. Stan Bynum. That system is based on the principles advocated earlier by Dr. Edward Howell (considered the discoverer of Enzyme Nutrition) and the patented research of Dr. Harvey Ashmead. It exploits the properties of amino acid mineral chelates to increase activity of a selective combination of different enzymes. The system is too complex to elaborate all the details here. Just a very brief outline should suffice.

Enzymes do require specific minerals like zinc, magnesium, cobalt, chromium, etc. as cofactors to reach their full activity. Soluble amino acid chelates maintain these minerals in a stable form to cross the intestinal wall, survive transport and participate in intracellular metabolism. Thus the system is known as CAeDS which is the acronym for Chelate-Activated enzyme Delivery System. The key patent (US# 4,863,898) is entitled "**Amino acid chelated compositions for delivery to specific biological tissue sites**". The CAeDS system is designed to impact each of the seven steps of cellular nutrition. Just the ideas illustrate the level of sophistication that researchers are now bringing to the design and application necessary to optimize the entire field of nutritional supplementation.

That brings us at last to the leading edge.

THE LEADING EDGE

That brief and selective lightning tour of the food supplement industry has brought us in time to the end of the 20th Century. The consumer market for these types of natural products has grown dramatically in the past 20 years, all across the Western World. In the US alone, total sales for dietary supplements were estimated at $4 billion in 1994, but that figure has now grown much larger to $27 billion in 2009 according to the trade journal, *Nutrition Business Journal.* Thousands of products have been offered for sale direct to the consumer in retail stores, health food outlets, nutrition centers and many pharmacies, as well as through network marketing distributors and via the internet. The actual number of dietary supplements on the market in the US has risen from approximately 4000 in 1994 to about 75,000 in 2008.

As the evolution of nutritional understanding and the consumer experience grows, still new products come on board every year. Then it seems that every few years some new product fundamentally expands the scope of nutritional practice by making advances in human physiology through careful research and clinical testing. Such breakthroughs are usually unpredictable and unexpected so they come about more often than not by mere serendipity. But when that happens, something novel and exciting promises to really make a significant difference to human health and wellbeing, if applied. So that enlightened horizon then becomes the leading edge of nutritional supplementation as the evolution continues.

How we got there at the dawn of this new century is the subject of the next chapter.

CHAPTER 5

Getting to the Leading Edge

This chapter tells a story – a rather dramatic story. It is a narrative that is as contemporary as today's news because it involves two of the hottest areas of mainstream research that have captured both public attention and professional excitement in the Western world. The application of emerging Stem Cell Technology is probably the most promising innovation for making major medical advances in the near future. Add to that the possibility of a new potential Bio-fuel that could, under optimum conditions produce 10-20 times more biomass per acre than ethanol derived from corn. That's an unlikely combination, but there you have it: Stem Cells and Bio-fuels – both as important today as any other field of inquiry.

What natural source could possibly impact both of these leading edge technologies and merit the attention of the best research minds in the world today? The answer is somewhat surprising. It is a product as ancient as the hills, and as common as the ubiquitous 'seaweed' found in salt and fresh water, whether in ponds, rivers, lakes or the wide open seas. But the term 'seaweed' is only appropriate when referring to the largest and most complex marine forms of a diverse group of organisms more generally referred to as algae (a term derived from the Latin for 'seaweed').

ALGAE SETS THE STAGE

Algae refers more generally then, to a very large group of simple photosynthetic organisms that range from single cells to huge multi-cellular forms like giant 'kelps' that can grow up to be 70 meters in length. Thousands of different species of algae have been identified and all research suggests that they were probably among the earliest life forms on earth. More importantly here, algae are at the bottom of the food chain. Microscopic forms that live suspended in the water column are called *phytoplankton* and they provide the essential food base in most marine food chains. Algae in its many forms is eaten by everything from the tiniest shrimp to the largest whales. In some ways they are the basis of all life on earth as we know it. They are capable of using combined nitrogen and of fixing carbon dioxide in the atmosphere to provide proteins, fats, oils, sugars … and obviously, energy.

Most attention has been given to the macro-algae (green algae), commonly described as seaweeds. These are an abundant source of nutrition and much, much more. However, most recently, the micro-algae or blue-green algae (including cyanobacteria) have come into the spotlight because they show some very interesting and intriguing properties with respect to their nutritive value. The latter category will become the focus of this book as we explore Stem Cell Nutrition more fully, but we cannot avoid mentioning here the historical applications of the macro –algae and the prospects for even more innovative developments in the future, as active research in this field continues.

People worldwide already use algae (generally macro-algae) in many ways. Most recently, the media focus has been largely on the possibilities of exploiting algae as an exceptional source for bio-fuel, in pursuit of green alternative energy. But for many years we have used algae to make fish food products, fertilizers, soil conditioners and livestock feed. It is also a fairly common source of alginates used in many food items like ice cream, serving as a thickening agent or stabilizer, etc. We've also used algae to treat sewage, thereby reducing the polluting effect of alternate toxic chemicals. Similarly, controlled algae can capture the undesirable fertilizers present in the runoff from typical farms, thereby improving the quality of water flowing into precious streams, rivers and finally oceans.

But all those applications pale in comparison to the potential nutritional value of algae for human consumption.

Expensive research on algae as a bio-fuel has waxed and waned in the West with the priorities of politicians, the risk tolerance of venture capitalists and the emergence of new challenges in implementation. At the same time, the search for other high-value algae products has intensified. Algae is now seen as a promising candidate to address major challenges of feeding the growing world population in the 21st century. For example, algae have been compared to the ever popular soybean. With year-round harvest opportunities, some algae can produce some 38 times more useable protein per acre per year than soy and just as importantly, it can be done with the use of just one percent of the fresh water that soy needs. That resulting algae protein, for example, can then be used in many food products, as well as in both animal and fish feed stocks. Just imagine the possibilities.

But that is all in the future. Right here and right now, algae (as a product - therefore we will use that as a singular term here) is already making its mark. It is a national food in several nations, especially in the Far East. The Chinese consume more than 70 species such as the vegetable '*fat choy*'; in Japan, over 20 species are common in the diet (including '*nori*' and '*aonori*'); in Ireland they use '*dulse*', while in Chile they use '*cochayayo.*' Add to these, '*laver*' in Wales, '*gim*' in Korea, and then 'sea lettuce' and '*badderlocks*' for salads in

Scotland, Ireland, Greenland and Iceland. Algae is fairly common in diets up and down the West coast of North America also (from California to British Columbia).

It is generally known that edible seaweeds are a good source of many vitamins including A, B1, B2, B6, niacin and C as well as a number of important minerals like iodine, potassium, iron, magnesium and calcium. Several algae varieties also provide essential fatty acids, especially the long-chain, essential omega-3 fatty acids. In fact, the fatty acids sought after in fish for all their health benefits originate in the oils of the micro-algae lower down the food chain.

We know that algae provide some rich sources of essential nutrients and we also know that there has been a long tradition of anecdotal evidence of health benefits associated with the safe consumption of edible algae (in many places and over many years). It is therefore not surprising that in the past few decades, commercially cultivated micro-algae including both the algae and its natural kin known as *cyanobacteria* (blue green algae), have been made available as nutritional supplements.

There are three noteworthy varieties of these micro-algae that have attracted most of the relatively new attention.

Spirulina is a free-floating filamentous cyanobacteria formally known as *Arthrospira*, usually found in tropical and subtropical lakes with low acidity. It has been used historically as a food source, but it is harvested commercially today mainly for use as a nutritional supplement around the world.

Chlorella is a single-cell green algae that has found its place in history as the plant originally studied to elucidate the mechanistic pathways of photosynthesis. It was once heralded as a promising primary food source and a possible solution to an earlier world hunger crisis.

But that turned out to have its own challenges and *chlorella* is popular today only as another nutritional supplement in fairly widespread use.

And now, here it comes …

***Aphanizomenon flos-aquae* (AFA)**, (Latin for 'Invisible Living Flower of the Water') is another unique fresh water species of blue-green algae. That brings us now to **the real superstar of this show.**

Did you hear the words 'lights, camera … action, just then? You should have, for what follows next is an amazing story of nature, science and human ingenuity. This was brought about not by clever and tedious investigation following some design, but rather by the coincidence of the right people, places and products that mysteriously fell into the right combination at the right time and in the right way. This is a true story of real serendipity.

Three characters perform the leading roles in this dramatic story. Let's meet the first of these.

ENTER CHRISTIAN DRAPEAU

Christian Drapeau was born in Montreal, Quebec in the mid-sixties. He grew up in that busy metropolis as a Canadian Francophone. That was just before the FLQ crisis and the confrontation with Prime Minister Pierre Elliot Trudeau; before the diminutive Premier of Quebec, Rene Levesque and the rising threat of separatism from Canada; before the two different failing referenda that turned that whole movement back on its heels.

Despite all the political excitement and upheaval going on around him, Christian remained rather shy and introspective as a young boy. But in his adolescent years he developed a love for reading and discovered an enchanting world in the French bookstores where he would go to browse for hours on end, several times a week. He vividly recalls that at age 14, he stumbled upon a particular book that seemed to describe 'the fantastic faculties of the brain.' He read about the work of the Bulgarian, Dr. Georgi Lozanov, a medical doctor who specialized in psychiatry and psychotherapy, but who also had a real passion for understanding how human beings learn.

Dr. Lozanov developed a new methodology of teaching and learning that enabled students to uncover 'the reserve capacities of the mind.' This accelerated learning technique allowed students to absorb subject matter at greatly increased rates. It drew international attention due to the remarkable success in the teaching of foreign languages. In general, students learned material several times faster with his new methodology than with 'normal' teaching methods. In 1975, Dr. Donald Schuster and Dr. Charles Gritton formed the Society for Accelerative Learning and Teaching (SALT) at Iowa State University. Soon this became a movement in the West and additional ideas were incorporated. Noted among these, Harvard Professor Howard Gardner developed a theory of *Multiple Intelligence*; Dr. Antonio Damasio demonstrated the critical importance of emotions in the learning process, while linguist John Grinder and psychologist Richard Bandler laid the foundations for *Neuro-Linguistic Programming*.

Young Christian got introduced to these ideas very early (recall, at about age 14) and he got hooked on them. He was constantly pouring over them in the bookstore and wanted so much to buy a few of these books and take them home. But he was intimidated because he thought his dad would not like this idea. However, he found a way to begin to apply what he was reading about. He had been training in *Tae Kwon Do* since he was only eight. When he was 15, The World Tae Kwon DO Federation announced the plan of having this martial art in demonstration at the 1984 Olympics in Los Angeles, hopefully to be later included for competition at the 1988 Games in Seoul. Christian was asked to compete in order to try to qualify for Team Canada. He was then a 'brown belt'. But after 7 years of rather intense training for such a young boy, his interest in martial art was slowly waning. He saw this as a great opportunity to test his newly acquired skills. He began training virtually every night, but not in a gym. He was training on his bed at home. He would spend hours using imagination and visualization techniques that he had learnt in a form of self hypnosis. He believed that this exercise programmed nerve pathways to allow him to execute his movements flawlessly in competition. He was proving for himself the power of his own mind. Christian went on to win the next North American competition as an 'acting black belt'. That dramatically boosted his self confidence and by the time he finished high school, he had become a self-assured purpose-driven young man, destined for greatness in some arena or another.

His fascination with the human brain was increasing exponentially. He read all he could about it in the encyclopedia and the more he read, the more questions he had and the more he just wanted to learn. He knew for sure that he wanted to pursue neurophysiology at university and McGill University was the only option for an undergraduate program in the field. That Honors program was restricted to just six students each year and he made the cut. Upon graduation he registered for post graduate research at the Montreal Neurological Institute associated with McGill, specializing in the area of epilepsy. As a young graduate student he was able to present a paper at the Second World Congress of NeuroScience in Budapest(1987).

But Christian Drapeau is no ordinary scientist. Even as a graduate student, his 'purist' ideals made him critical of research methodology and the ready acceptance of scientific dogma. One day the Dean of the Faculty took umbrage with his bold critique of a theory about phantom limbs developed by Ronald Melzack – then a professor at

McGill - and upbraided him: "Why don't you wait until you have your PhD before you start having your own opinions!" Christian never forgot those words. He became increasingly disillusioned with his research environment. He was in search of truth and concluded he was in the wrong arena. So he made a move – a dramatic move. He took all the work developed under his PhD program and wrote a Master's thesis. He then went off to France to study Comparative Religion in a monastery there. Six months later, he received a letter requesting that more work be done to complete his Master's thesis and returned to McGill. He was content to tidy up the research he had already done and complete the Master's program with a thesis and get out. That he did.

Christian did not return to the monastery as he had planned. Instead, he began to pursue the earlier passion for accelerated learning, especially after he met a friend who was really struggling with repetitive learning and was getting nowhere. He developed an original workshop to exploit all the insights and methodologies he was gaining in that field. In fact, back at age 19, Christian had already put them to work in a practical way by learning to speak fluent English (a prerequisite to study at McGill) in just a few weeks. He then qualified for the Honors Program. With this new learning methodology, he knew he was on to something with great potential and usefulness. So after completing his Masters degree, he developed an original workshop to help teachers to teach and students to learn more efficiently and effectively. The workshop first became a manual and later a book, '*J'apprends à aprendre*' (literally in English, 'I learn to learn'), which has been translated into six other languages. In fact that book was selected by UNESCO as one of two hundred texts recommended internationally for educators. In a nutshell, it is designed to help students learn how to manage information in order to produce faster learning.

All this would later become very useful when Christian started travelling and speaking around the world. After a lecture in Puerto Rico where he had to use a translator, he made the commitment that he would learn Spanish in order to more effectively share his message in Hispanic countries. He went to Costa Rica, at the ILISA School, and worked 1-on-1 with a teacher. On the fifth day he gave a lecture on stem cells to the medical students at the University of Costa Rica! "That was the most mentally draining experience of my entire life," he shared. In a similar way, he managed to teach himself music and learned to play the guitar. He had learned early in his life that the brain had an amazing capacity that far exceeded normal expectations and he presupposed that all things were indeed possible, to those who would learn to tap that amazing human potential.

Christian Drapeau was only getting started.

One day he was invited to a presentation in Montreal and the main subject considered was destined to become the superstar of this narrative, but at that time there were neither 'lights and drums', nor even 'bells and whistles'. The whole event was somewhat low key, with an emphasis on anecdotal reporting. There was little science to impress him and no persuasive factual evidence to convince him. Christian listened attentively but at the end of the presentation, he was more intrigued by the subject matter than he was impressed with the rather poor presenter. He followed up by doing some reading about this amazing 'blue-green algae called AFA' that was being reported by several attendees to have remarkable health benefits. Most interesting to Christian was the anecdotal accounts of effects on the brain – rekindling his passion for that field once again. Among other benefits, consumers had been reporting anecdotal experiences of improved mood, overall increase in mental alertness and stamina, short and long term memory, problem solving, creativity, recall of dreams, a heightened sense of wellbeing and sharper focus. This type of language was to Christian like honey is to bees. He was fascinated once again. The more he learned about AFA even then, as relatively primitive as the understanding was at that time, the more he became intrigued and motivated. As he began reading more he was convinced that the case for AFA was not being given justice by the presenters he had listened to. He knew soon after, that he could do a much better job and he had the audacity to suggest no less.

Given his first opportunity in Montreal not long after this first meeting, he became an instant hit with his surprised audience. One thing led to another and soon he was in demand, giving evening lectures and then all day seminars to AFA distributors, consumers and anyone interested enough to listen. With his ultra fast learning curve being accelerated, he was soon the 'local expert' on AFA in Quebec.

Word spread further afield and by the following year (1994) he was addressing the major Annual Convention of the parent company responsible for the AFA activity in Quebec at that time. Again, Christian was so dynamic and impressive at the convention, the company arranged for him to speak three or four times a year thereafter. But that soon escalated. He gave 26 lectures in the first five months of 1995 all over North America. Almost every weekend he was speaking somewhere and his subject matter had now expanded beyond just AFA. He was lecturing on antioxidants like CoQ10, probiotics, digestive enzymes and more. In a short time, Christian had mastered the background material on many aspects of nutritional supplements, natural products in general, herbal medicine and other alternative therapies. He was fascinated just consuming and digesting all this new exciting material that seemed to be so relevant and to make so much common sense. He knew then that he had been introduced to something big but he just did not appreciate how big it could really become.

Within a year of that first annual convention speech, the owners of the company came to recognize Christian's vast knowledge of the industry (so rapidly acquired) and his other amazing talents. They therefore asked him to become their Director of Research and Development. He accepted. He was given a $1 million budget to develop a proper Quality Control Department for the company and to initiate some original research to further substantiate the true value of AFA.

Christian Drapeau was no Anthony Robbins. But given the opportunity, he was growing by leaps and bounds. He had become an excellent speaker – confident, compelling and in demand. But it was his message and the science behind his supposed propositions on stage that had much more room to grow. He needed more exposure to science and to mainstream research to justify what he was perceiving so instinctively. In this new position in R & D, he could reach out to collaborate once again with research professionals. Only this time, he was not a student anymore, no longer at the Montreal Neurological Institute or McGill. Rather, he was now free to have his own opinions and ideas. He now had some significant research dollars to deploy and he quickly realized that 'Whoever pays the piper, calls the tune.'

This was the beginning of what would become a wide collaboration with other scientists in different universities and research centers. He would go on to coauthor many articles for publication in the scientific literature over the next fifteen years and beyond. No other collegial collaboration would prove more vital or valuable than the one he established with Dr. Gitte Jensen. None of his publications would prove as seminal as the hypothesis they would later put forward together in Medical Hypothesis 2002, entitled "The Use of insitu Bone Marrow Stem Cells for the Treatment of various Degenerative Diseases"[1].

But we must first meet this second star of our unfolding drama.

ENTER DR. GITTE JENSEN

Dr. Jensen is quite a contrast to Christian Drapeau. She is a brilliant, soft spoken lady who has always been a scientist at heart. Born in Denmark, she grew up surrounded by a community immersed in alternative health approaches but with little science substantiation. She felt a growing desire to acquire skills to help put scientific evaluation behind solid modalities for health and preventive medicine, and to help weed out what could not be scientifically substantiated. She attended the University of Aarhus in the 1980's where she obtained her Doctorate in Immunology and Microbiology. After further post-doctoral work in Denmark, she moved to the University of Alberta in Edmonton to continue research in her chosen field. In a later move to Montreal, she was appointed as Assistant Professor in the Department of Surgery at McGill University and maintained her research laboratory at the Royal Victoria Hospital Research Institute.

Christian did not know Dr. Jensen while at McGill. He had actually left before she arrived. However, their introduction was more than fortuitous. Dr. Jensen had started questioning her rather narrow academic path, and was seeking research opportunities to get back to her roots of why she started her education, namely to seek the truth about nutritional, herbal and unorthodox healthy interventions. By strange coincidence, a friend of hers had introduced her earlier to the AFA product that was the subject of anecdotal reports related to   relief of many chronic health problems. She hypothesized that the immune system was at the core of this improved well-being. Another aspect of interest was the reported effects of AFA on mental focus and mood, which was later to become an additional focus of her research with Christian Drapeau.

That led to an arranged meeting of these two brilliant minds. Christian Drapeau, then a   Director of R & D, with his knowledge of AFA, natural products (including herbs) and other alternative therapies, on the one hand, was now connected to Dr. Gitte Jensen, the immunologist who was well equipped to do advanced pre-clinical and clinical research at McGill University and who was also intrigued by the possibly active ingredients and mode(s) of action of these blue-green algae derivatives, on the other. Thus, began a relationship of synergistic collaboration that would see them emerge at the leading edge of nutritional supplementation where the science is today.

Dr. Jensen took AFA to her McGill laboratory and did preliminary experiments where she found effects on different immune system cells *in vitro*. She then committed with Christian and together they spent several months developing a research proposal. It involved recruiting 50 people over the course of several years - 25 volunteers consuming AFA, plus 25 others consuming placebo. Of course, none of the volunteers would know what they were taking. The subjects would each take orally 2 x 250mg of the blue green algae, three times a day for up to three months. They would also have blood taken at 0, 2 weeks and 3 months. The scientists would test their blood for a very wide range of cell parameters and analyze the data in double blind fashion to see what effects could be observed. This was a huge undertaking, since the processing of one person's blood sample involved a full laboratory day for three skilled technicians.

At first, there was complete disappointment. There was no significant difference in the results seen with either group - not control or placebo. None whatsoever! *Rien du tout!* That's often the course of even good research. Someone has well said that *'if you know everything about what you're doing and so your results are predictable, then you're not doing research'*. All technology in fact advances down the corridor of disappointment and failure. By the process of necessary elimination, one arrives at solutions, unravels the answers one seeks and discovers ultimately, the success that's deserved. Perhaps, that's how it should be. Someone else said that 'if wishes were horses, then all beggars would ride', and in a similar way, if technology was predictable then breakthroughs would come daily. But they don't. Each one demands the courage to try, the resilience to try again and yes, the persistence to never give up.

Dr. Jensen and Christian Drapeau did not give up - of course not. They were not only clear thinkers, they were also being good scientists and researchers. They had reason to hope, even though there were no differences observed in both subjects and controls (blinded by design of course) after the first few months of their investigation. Could this be an exercise in futility? Did the algae really do anything? Perhaps a brainstorming session would help.

'Double blind studies' imply that both the researchers and the subjects do not know which is 'placebo' or which is 'control'. In that sense everyone was coded. A nervous Christian broke the code himself and came up empty. There was nothing to report. No change, no trend, no effect observed. Brainstorm again - and again. Could it be that the effect was very transient and not noticeable after weeks?

It was back to the drawing board - but not exactly. The immune system is geared to kick into action immediately upon encountering a threat to health. What if it was the timing of the blood draws that had been based on a more mainstream thinking of 'nutritional loading'? Rather, could it not otherwise be a rapid effect caused – not by nutrient(s) in the classical sense – but by highly bioactive substances with very specific effects in the body? In pursuit of an answer, they decided to use similar protocols as before, but this time they would draw blood at time 0, 30, 60, 120 minutes. If they missed it, they would really miss it … but what if they caught it?! And they did catch it! There was a clear change in the number of Natural Killer (NK) cells seen in the peripheral blood soon after the algae was consumed, which was interpreted as an increase in the migration of NK Cells out of the blood into tissues. That was the first positive indication that something was happening. It was small, but it opened a floodgate of possibilities now waiting to be further investigated.

A key question that readily comes to the mind of an immunologist or just any scientist would be -- what is the active ingredient? Concomitant work done at the University of Mississippi, coordinated by Christian and funded by his employer, had recently demonstrated that a polysaccharide fraction of AFA extract showed enhancement of NK cell activity following administration for seven days[2]. Dr. Jensen was able to show in her laboratory that the polysaccharide fraction of the AFA she was working with was also responsible for the effect on NK cell migration, as well as the stimulation of immune cell mobilization and macrophage activation[3]. She later demonstrated that AFA also stimulated NK cell activation[4].

The former part of this research was all happening just before Y2K. That was leading up to the year 2000 and the start of the new millennium. That was a time of anticipated global change. But local change was also in the air ... for both Christian Drapeau and Dr. Jensen.

First, Christian was about to make a major move. He knew why, but he did not know where. The 'why' related to the company he was involved with. He had become the face of confidence and credibility to the host of field distributors and consumers who relied on his knowledge and expertise, as well as his caring and common touch. The company had run into financial problems. Apparently it had begun to engage in some rather questionable if not unethical practices. It was fighting government agencies to defend itself against accusations of misrepresentation and unjustifiable medical claims. There was internal squabbling and family discord among the principals of the company. Added to that, was a tug-o-war with the field in that people felt cheated by the company and its owner. All this and more left Christian with only Hobson's choice. He had no choice but to resign and this he did honorably just after returning from a lecture in Boulder, Colorado where the last straw broke the camel's back. He had seen enough, he had done enough and now he had had enough. He slammed that door behind him, uncertain of his next steps. However, he felt real good doing just that.

As fate would have it, he did not have long to wait. By coincidence again, soon after, he was passing through an airport, when he ran into an acquaintance he had known through his involvement with algae and the ecology of the lake region in which it was harvested. The small airport sees some 10-20,000 people go through each year but on this particular day, just after Y2K, here comes Christian Drapeau, unassuming and unannounced, intersecting the path of the third star of our unfolding drama. His name is Howard Newman.

ENTER HOWARD NEWMAN

Howard Newman is not a scientist at all but a shrewd successful entrepreneur and businessman. He has some forty years of experience in aquaculture, and specifically the harvesting and distribution of *zooplankton* (the tiny creatures that occupy the bottom of the aquatic food chains). In contrast to phytoplankton (*phyto*: 'plant' and *plankton*: 'wanderer' or 'drifter') which we met earlier, zooplankton refers to animal species. They are sometimes too small to see with the naked eye but they drift everywhere in water – fresh water ponds, lakes, rivers and in the open seas and oceans. To Howard Newman, they represent a gold mine. He has a long track record in the USA brine shrimp (*Artemia*) industry.

Artemia are interesting aquatic crustaceans that go back possibly millions of years but appear to have remained unchanged. They are at best about half-an-inch in size and have three eyes and eleven pairs of legs (who knows why?). They actually circulate hemoglobin in their blood. Amazing. Their thick-shelled eggs (cysts) are stable for years – apparently, even centuries! - and will still hatch when placed in water. Imagine that. In nature, they favor salt-water lakes and are rare in the open sees. They swim upside down because ... ? Any guess would be as good as any other. Those exotic little creatures were Howard Newman's first business interest. It is said that he has probably been knee deep in more Artemia lakes than anyone in the world!

From 1970 to 1984 Howard owned and managed *Artemia Inc.* which harvested *Artemia* from the Great Salt Lake in Utah and Shack Bay in Australia. The company also imported cysts from Brazil and manufactured both as fish food. Howard Newman saw opportunity where others only saw slime, scum and slush or even did not see anything at all. He successfully transformed his small harvesting operation into a multi-million dollar company selling fish food.

Then, from 1984 to 1990, Howard was Vice-President of *San Francisco Bay Brands*, the primary provider of *Artemia* to the reptile and tropical fish markets. In 1990, Bay Brands was purchased by *INVE* and he stayed with INVE for ten subsequent years as the Executive Manager for the Americas. During that time he was instrumental in increasing the company's sales to over $20 million annually. *INVE Aqua culture* is the worldwide leader in *Artemia* products, based in Belgium since 1983, and today remains the premier global supplier of shrimp hatchery feeds.

In 1999, Howard directed the consolidation of the aquaculture industry in Utah, where he negotiated and completed the strategic alliance of eight competitors, thereby eliminating a lot of duplication of services and allowing INVE to spearhead the sales and marketing efforts.

By March of 2000, Mr. Newman took on a new challenge. He and his son Gregory, (together they own a privately held company, *Desert Lake Technologies*) acquired *Rossha Enterprises Inc.* This latter company had been in business since 1984, harvesting, processing and marketing AFA grown naturally in one of the largest lakes in the Pacific Northwest of the United States. But Howard's interest was not AFA. He was in fact, interested in a small zooplankton living in the lake alongside AFA. This was *Daphnia pulicaria*. They acquired Rossha in order to have the equipment to harvest Daphnia.

Daphnia are also interesting little creatures themselves. They are even smaller than *Artemia*, growing typically no more than half of the latter's size. They live in various aquatic environments, ranging from acidic swamps to freshwater lakes and streams. They have a translucent carapace covering most of their body, so under the microscope one can observe the eye moving, the heart beating, and blood flowing. What a treat for the eyes. They also produce robust eggs that survive under harsh environmental conditions. They are a popular live food for tropical and marine fish – a market industry in its own right.

When Christian and Howard ran into each other that day at the airport, they were quick to catch up on each other's interests and current activities. They had met two or three times before but then they were both inhabiting different spaces. But timing is everything. They were both prepared for this encounter, so they spoke differently, they listened attentively and they heard exactly what they wanted to hear. Howard had recently acquired his new company prospect, with plans to make it grow, and Christian had just left his own hopeful enterprise behind. Christian was disillusioned and disappointed but not despairing. Howard was enterprising and engaged with much excitement, but in need of expert help.

In fact, they needed each other. Howard was focused on harvesting more Daphnia from the nearby lake while Christian was still fascinated by the other big scientific (even if not commercial) prospect on the lake – and for Christian himself that prospect was still nothing else but AFA. When Christian shared his growing enthusiasm for AFA with Howard just one month after leaving the fiasco of his previous company, he jokingly (but hopefully) advanced an immediate proposition. If Howard could make a profitable business from harvesting and marketing Daphnia, why could Christian not take up the challenge and develop the market for Daphnia's harvesting by-product, AFA? Christian was quick to point out that after all, AFA was probably the first food on earth, with a robust DNA that made it an invaluable 'life force', an entirely natural product derived from a pristine environment. He was being somewhat prophetic, but without knowing it.

The Drapeau proposal was not about fish food like Howard's Daphnia was intended. He was talking about feeding humans – yes, humans with a food supplement that he had come to believe would surpass all expectations when the research uncovered its true potential. He recounted the early results coming out of Dr. Jensen's Laboratory at McGill in Montreal.

So, here came Christian's closing argument. He could re-brand AFA and promote *Desert Lake Technologies* that Howard was so anxious to put on the industrial map…. as a Biotech company. That had the right sound and the right feel but it would now have the right product. Imagine AFA with active ingredients shown to produce positive biological results including anti-inflammatory effects from phycocyanin[5]. Then there were central nervous system enhancements from a molecule called phenylethylamine (PEA),[6] as well as the immune-enhancing effects on NK cells and macrophages from the polysaccharide component[3,4]. At that time, the benefits associated with PEA seemed to be the most relevant and promising of all.

Why? It was the timing again.

For some time before that, three herbal products had been widely acclaimed in the alternative therapy/herbal medicine community. Many consumers had been taking supplements containing Kava, Ma Huang (Ephedra) or St. John's Wort which all traditionally had mood enhancing properties and increased energy and focus. People seemed to feel better, period. That was until reports of possible toxicity (to liver and kidneys)[7] hit the media and the inevitable happened. The reports were all later challenged[8] but the market damage was immediate. Several products were banned and consumer confidence was shaken.

So if Howard was persuaded, the market was already open just at that time. AFA would come to the market with great promise to fill that void and with a clean track record for safety and a compelling story as Christian had already summarized in his spontaneous pitch to him.

Howard was sold. Christian was excited. The deal was done. Right there - Right then! So in March of 2000, Christian joined Desert Lake Technologies. He made his move. He changed his plans to return to Canada, obtained new work permits so he could stay in the United States and soon got down to business.

That was Christian Drapeau's turn of events. What about Dr. Jensen? Was she on the move too?

Yes, she was.

Back at McGill Dr. Jensen felt increasingly stifled in the academic environment where a narrow path was strongly encouraged, and a serious scientific interest in overall health considered too broad a topic for scientific pursuit.

Dr. Jensen is a true researcher at heart. That's her passion and that's all she really wanted to do - then and now. In 1998, she set up a private research corporation focused on integrative health research and communication. In addition, the idea grew of starting a private laboratory where there would be a well-defined focus for customized scientific research protocols, developed specifically to provide science-based claims-support for the natural products industry. This all made good sense.

Christian loved the idea. He persuaded Howard to have Desert Lake Technologies initially support the new research laboratory and Dr. Jensen was ready to make her move. She left McGill in 2000 and moved with her family to Oregon. *Natural Immune Systems* (known today as *NIS Labs*) the new contract research laboratory was born, with Dr. Gitte Jensen as Research Director.

The result of all this was that in 2000, the three stars of our drama were now finally all on the same stage. They were brought together by the hands of fate as the choice players in an unfolding story, still undetermined but somehow anticipated to become very significant. Christian was at Desert Lake Technologies anxious to explore the science of AFA and then to justify and communicate the health benefits to be derived by human consumption. At the same time, Dr. Jensen was now in her own laboratory ready to do what she has always loved best. She would continue to do research *in vitro* and *in vivo* on cell-based physiological phenomena impacted by natural products. AFA would be her Exhibit A. Meanwhile, Howard Newman had DLT up and running, harvesting not only his long-time friend and focus – that is Daphnia – but also anticipating something new and wonderful to happen. He now had scientists on his team who just could, in principle, discover something more to revolutionize the industry to which he has devoted most of his life. They were all primed and rearing to go, as Y2K announced the birth of a new millennium with all the hope, possibility and promise of the future.

A NEW HYPOTHESIS

So everybody got down to the business at hand. Christian got busy applying his accelerated learning techniques to review the scientific literature. He read many papers about immune modulation and anti-inflammatory mechanisms; about neurotransmitters and CNS effects of natural products; about traditional uses of AFA, etc., etc. There was so much out there to absorb. Meanwhile, Dr. Jensen was busy setting up her new laboratory, hiring new staff, writing research proposals, soliciting contract research, etc., etc. At the same time, Howard Newman was being the good businessman, looking for improvements for harvesting and processing his Daphnia and blue-green-algae, while of course, seeking out new markets.

It did not take long for a breakthrough to take place. Christian was fascinated and puzzled by the wide diversity of symptomatic benefit that consumers of AFA had traditionally reported. He knew first hand of people who demonstrated real benefits that he could not explain. Either this blue green algae – *'nature's first food'*, he recalled – had such a variety of active ingredients to have such an effect on different organs, physiological mechanisms and systems in the human body, or perhaps some specific ingredient(s) was doing something more fundamental.

Dr. Jensen was encouraged by the science that had come out of the clinical studies at McGill – namely, the demonstration of rapid and transient effects after AFA consumption. However, she kept thinking that the major core player had been missed. The immune cells alone could not adequately account for all the profound effects of AFA, such as nerve system rejuvenation, recovery from trauma and increased pancreatic function in diabetics. She kept digging into the literature to increase the understanding of underlying mechanisms.

During a sabbatical in her undergraduate supervisor's laboratory back in Denmark, she had done work on hematopoietic stem cells, primarily in cancer patients undergoing bone marrow stem cell transplants. It was therefore natural that she kept her eye on the stem cell literature, even though at that time, stem cells were of peripheral importance beyond the hematopoietic system. At the end of the year 2000, she came across a newly published article that changed her outlook o the reported effects of AFA. The article was entitled, "Turning Blood into Brain ..." (9) She got on the phone with Christian Drapeau and was somewhat miffed when the first ten minutes of the call were drowned in Christian's laughter. She was only focused on the scientific discovery – namely, that hematopoietic stem cells were found to have much broader potential for regeneration of multiple tissues and organs. Christian however, found it immensely humorous that the discovery had only been made based on injection of male stem cells into female mice, and the tracking of the Y chromosome in female brains. (If you did not laugh yourself just then, you probably would if you think again about it – that really is funny, though perhaps a bit subtle.)

Gitte had some talking to do to convince Christian that indeed the regeneration associated with the stem cells was not a simple effect of a 'tiny little Y chromosome' ...

When the laughter subsided, both agreed that this had immense potential. Stem cell support might be the unifying factor for many of the observations associated with consumption of AFA. But what was the active compound? Gitte already found it was the high molecular weight polysaccharide fraction of AFA that impacted these cells. But what to make of all the anecdotal evidence for a wide variety of health benefits to some people who suffered from such diverse conditions? One particular woman's story had haunted Christian more than any other. She was a 60 year old who had suffered third degree burns nearly 50 years ago. When she took AFA, after one year there was little evidence of any scarring on her skin and she showed him the pictures to prove it. He was not in denial, he was really puzzled and rightly so.

Then Christian started to read extensively about stem cells. Remember this is just after Y2K. President George Bush had just come through a tough and tight election campaign where the issue of government funding of embryonic stem cell (ESC) research was hotly debated. Recall speeches at the Democratic Convention in Los Angeles promising potential cures that could be found using this ESC approach for major, chronic debilitating illnesses like Parkinson's, ALS or Alzheimer's and even fatal diseases. Pro-life activists would have none of it. It posed a serious ethical dilemma and Americans were divided on this issue for sure. Then President Bush made a ruling in 2001 limiting the further use of new human embryos to derive any more ESC lines. Stem cells were very prominent in the news at that time. There was ever so much excitement and controversy in the media, but the focus later proved to be misguided.

Christian Drapeau kept reading the literature. He was intrigued by recent research papers that showed how adult bone marrow cells could give rise to different cell types in different organs including the brain, the heart, muscle tissue, liver tissue and so on.

Soon the new NIS Laboratory would find another source of funding locally. It came from the Jeld-Wen Foundation, a charitable arm of the widely successful *Jeld-Wen Company*. This company had transformed from a small Oregon millwork plant in the 1960s with just 15 employees, into a worldwide operation of over 20,000 employees producing windows and doors, second to none. The foundation is a private, non-profit organization created in 1969 to invest in worthy projects in communities where the company operates. They have contributed to hundreds of endeavours, including schools, colleges, hospitals, museums and neighbourhood centers. Jeld-Wen's founder and CEO, Richard (Dick) Wendt was actually a user/consumer of

AFA and that certainly influenced this grant in support of Dr. Jensen's research on AFA at NIS.

Dick Wendt was a strong facilitator and a handshake kind of guy. He was a great and positive influence and demonstrated that one only achieves by stopping the chatter and putting one foot in front of the other. His quiet presence infused people around him as soon as he entered the room, and the example he set – and expected of everyone around him – was that of proper conduct. He would keep his word, and expected everyone else to follow through with similar straightforward simplicity and transparency. He was a man of integrity and possessed a royal old-fashioned sense of honor.

His interest in health at all levels (both personal and community health) and his scientific curiosity made it a privilege for anyone in this field to know him and work with him. The lack of evidence of a public ego on his part was a key influence on moving these projects forward. Although Dick Wendt seemed to shun the spotlight, the evidence of the seeds he and his wife Nancy planted and nurtured are evidenced in the local community. Although Dick Wendt did not see the final success of the projects he strongly supported, his concepts of personal responsibility and sustainability continues to infuse them.

Gitte and Christian were now full of new ideas and idealism, but without the solid support from Dick Wendt this story may never have moved this far or this fast. Yet, that the story did. The quiet, stubborn years from 2000 to 2002 proved to be a test of fortitude and persistence. It was a slow and tedious process – a long circuitous path along which these two devoted scientists tried to convince themselves that what they were perceiving – slowly but surely – was indeed correct. They had to establish to their full satisfaction that the data they were collecting was solid. That was time-consuming, painstaking and expensive research. In fact, the final proofs, including clinical studies, were only made possible through the unwavering support of Dick Wendt. That found its fullest expression when Desert Lake Technologies and the local Merle West Center for Medical Research (a non-profit research organization, where Dick Wendt served as Chairman of the Board) came together to form a new partnership known as Lake Algae Research. This partnership led to a solid plan, sufficient funding and an on-going process of due diligence that facilitated the breakthroughs they anticipated.

Eventually success did come. Slowly the truth emerged. If NK cell mobilization is stimulated by AFA, since NK cells and stem cells are in the same lineage of "white blood cells', could it just be possible that somehow AFA might stimulate stem cell mobilization too? Coincidentally, Dr. Jensen had the capability of putting the novel idea to the test. She led her group back to the laboratory to carefully design and execute the clinical trial to test this really provocative idea. They did so and after checking and rechecking the raw data they were driven to only one conclusion ... **EUREKA!** ... In summary, the **AFA was demonstrated to increase stem cell populations in the peripheral blood of humans, soon after it was consumed**[10].

They repeated the assays just to be sure. Here's what Dr. Jensen's team did. Healthy human volunteers were identified and the proportion of CD34+ cells that was circulating in the peripheral blood of each subject was evaluated prior to consumption of AFA and then hourly for up to four (4) hours after consumption. (Recall that CD34+ is a good marker for stem cells). The volunteers were instructed to limit physical and mental activity for a time, before and after consumption of AFA. Each person was provided 5gm of dried AFA. Red blood cells in whole blood samples from each volunteer were lysed in a standard solution to remove them. The remaining cells were washed and stained with monoclonal antibody carrying a fluorescein conjugate. Samples were fixed in formalin and analyzed by flow cytometry. The net results showed a peak (25% increase) in circulating CD34+ cells at about 2-3 hours after consumption, compared to controls. By four hours after ingestion of AFA, the circulating CD34+ cells returned to their baseline value. The net summary was that AFA can enhance the release of endogenous (adult) stem cells from the bone marrow (and possibly other anatomical sites) directly into the blood circulation. **Consumption of AFA mobilizes CD34+ stem cells.**

Now let's follow the logic of the development closely. From what the reader will recall about stem cells from Part One, stem cells also have characteristic markers for adhesion and homing to specific tissues. More specifically the L-selectin (CD62L) surface molecule (receptor) favours 'homing', i.e. the 'sensing involved in the decision-making for a cell when it either stays at a location or moves on. Other markers (such as CD11b and CD11c) influence adhesion, like glue, but only come into play after a decision is made. When we discuss stem cells, L-selectin is of double importance: The receptor is involved in the decision of whether a stem cell stays in the bone marrow where it was made, or whether it moves on in search of something to fix. Once the stem cell is on the move, L-selectin is also involved in the decision the stem cell makes about whether and when to 'home' into a tissue in need of repair. The question was then: do the CD34+ stem cells which are mobilized into circulation when AFA is consumed, express the same adhesion molecules?

Following on this, Dr. Jensen's team could do assays for the specific cell surface molecules before and after AFA consumption. They were quick to demonstrate that the mobilized CD34+ cells retained the same adhesion and homing phenotype after AFA ingestion, indicating that the cells had normal ability to 'home'.

Christian Drapeau could hardly contain himself. He began to put the pieces together. He had discovered that several recent publications addressing the same stem cell issue had concluded - unequivocally - that stem cells from the bone marrow can migrate and populate multiple distant tissues. This had been demonstrated with two principal techniques. In the first, bone marrow from male mice donors (carrying the Y chromosome) was injected into previously irradiated female mice (of course sub lethally, not enough to kill them). Bone marrow stem cells could then be stimulated in the female recipients by injecting G-CSF. Samples of blood and various cell and tissue samples (after selective sacrificing of the animals over time) would then be examined for the presence of the Y chromosome. The positive tests for the Y chromosome would then indicate that these cells originated from the bone marrow cells of the male donor. The test used could detect either Hy antigen immuno fluorescence or the fluorescence seen after in situ hybridization, using probes for the Y chromosome[11].

In the second technique, bone marrow cells from the transgenic male donor mice were labelled with the green fluorescent protein (GFP) and injected again into irradiated isogenic female mice recipients. The animals were all treated as before and the subsequent blood and tissue types (just as before) were examined for the expression of GFP using flow cytometry. This again, indicated donor origin.

Clearly, in the literature there was evidence that bone marrow stem cells were trafficking under these conditions. The injected cells were homing, implanting and differentiating into multiple distant tissue types. There was conclusive evidence for bone marrow stem cells becoming cells of the brain, muscle, heart, liver and more. But the mindset remained on the process of intervention. If one *injected* stem cells or if one used G-CSF like a *drug* to stimulate their release from the bone marrow, *then* and by implication *only then* did this phenomenon arise. Clinicians, it seemed, had to do something. So they thought. That is the usual medical mindset.

However, Christian Drapeau reflected on all this and then brainstormed with Dr. Jensen. The pieces were coming together, slowly but surely. If a natural product like AFA supported stem cell release, might there not be a natural even spontaneous release of stem cells from the bone marrow? Why not? … **EUREKA!!** -- for the second time. A new hypothesis was conceived. Here it comes.

In situ mobilization of stem cells from the bone marrow and their migration to different tissues is a normal *physiological process* of regeneration and repair. Possible therapeutic benefits can be generated with less invasive regimens than the removal and re-injection of stem cells, through the natural *stimulation* of normal stem cell mobilization and migration(1).

The pair of stem cell visionaries got down to work with a new sense of urgency. They had a bright idea and they knew it. After all the media excitement and publicity about embryonic stem cells and the miraculous cures that had been conceived, perhaps everyone else had been missing the woods for the trees. Here was a fundamental renewal system of nature and the human body in particular, that had been overlooked by so many and for so long. The spontaneous release of stem cells from the bone marrow and the recruitment and homing of those cells from the circulation appears to be a normal aspect of human physiology.

This was a remarkable idea, especially at that time. Just reflect that stem cell research had got to the point then where the media, the researchers by and large, and the general public had come to think of stem cells and possibly stem cell therapy as something derived mainly from fetuses or at least something involving the removal of cells from the body, then culturing and freezing for later re-injection. What a contrast to think now of stem cells as intrinsic in origin, ubiquitous in distribution and continuously active – personally. As the mantra for this book expresses it:

Everybody has stem cells; everybody uses stem cells; everybody uses stem cells everyday; stem cells work and ... they work every time.

There was so much more to be done now. Dr. Jensen and Christian Drapeau had to tidy up all the loose ends of the research protocols and data analysis. Next, they had to prepare patent applications for submission, to protect these ideas which could have significant commercial implications. Then all these ideas were drafted into a manuscript and submitted for publication. The year 2001 was a busy one indeed.

The first provisional patent application was filed on May 14 of that year. The resulting **Patent No: US 6,814,961 B1** was later issued to the inventors: Gitte S. Jensen and Christian Drapeau on November 9, 2004 with the descriptive title:

'Method for Enhancing Stem Cell Trafficking.'

ABSTRACT: **'Consumption of blue-green algae or extracts thereof, enhances trafficking or homing of stem cells in animals by inducing a transient increase in the population of stem cells present in the animal's circulatory system. The animal may be healthy or suffering some disease or physiological condition.'**

This patent, assigned to Desert Lake Technologies, included as evidence for claim, two remarkable case reports. It may be useful to point out that Case Reports in science are of some value, especially in breaking new research ground. They are never conclusive by themselves, but they certainly illustrate what's practically possible. They open the mind to think creatively, outside the conventional box, and to be receptive to something new. Many a breakthrough in science originated with the observation of something unusual, a result that did not fit existing paradigms.

The first *Case Report* was of a 65 year old male with a long history of a mildly compromised immune system (with recurrence of symptomatic chicken pox, five times during childhood) and inflammatory conditions during adulthood, including arthritis. He demonstrated tissue repair in multiple body locations within about two weeks after beginning consumption of 1.5 gm AFA per day. Tissue repair occurred in muscle and dermal tissue on the forehead, lower back and right knee. The knee and back were sites of prior surgery at ages 15 and 45, respectively. The subject had suffered tissue damage to his forehead resulting from a car accident at age 25. This latter injury included an abundance of small glass splinters embedded in the skin and muscle of the forehead. After two weeks of regular AFA consumption, and approximately 40 years after his forehead injury occurred, about 30 small lesions formed on the subject's forehead, each containing a glass splinter! Once the glass splinters were expelled, the area healed with no further scarring. Unbelievable - but true!

The second *Case Report* was of a 52 year old female with a history of severe allergies and fibromyalgia. She was observed over a four year period while consuming 1.5g AFA per day for the first three years, and larger quantities during the fourth year. Observations of clinical symptoms of allergies, intense muscle pain associated with fibromyalgia, and microbial forms associated with red blood cells were conducted. [A correlation exists between parasitized red blood cells and fibromyalgia/chronic fatigue syndrome]. Over the four year period of observations, consumption of AFA increased the subject's tolerance to foods that previously initiated an anaphylactic reaction. AFA consumption also correlated with an increased proportion of non-parasitized versus parasitized red blood cells, thus improving delivery of oxygen to muscle tissue and reducing muscle pain. It seems that AFA consumption stimulated hematopoietic cells to produce more red blood cells.

By November of that same year, the manuscript for publication had also been prepared. The Drapeau/Jensen team had refined their ideas and *therefore submitted to Medical Hypotheses Journal, the original seminal paper entitled:* '***The Use of*** in situ **Bone Marrow Stem Cells for the treatment of various Degenerative Diseases.**'[1] Having established that the consumption of AFA, a naturally occurring edible product, can enhance the release and trafficking of stem cells from the bone marrow, they went on to propose that 'efforts should be made to identify other natural compounds characterized by their ability to augment this normal process … for the potential treatment of various degenerative diseases.'

But a looming question remained, like the big elephant in the room. What active ingredient(s) in AFA might be responsible for the stem cell effects observed and perhaps more so, what possible mechanism(s) might be involved? That's basic to science. 'What' and 'How' should always be specific, if an understanding or any degree of control of the phenomenon was to be realized. Therein was the major challenge still ahead.

SERENDIPITY

Where does one begin to look for an active ingredient in a natural product - especially with limited funds for research? At least in this instance, there was an obvious starting point. It was already known that high molecular weight polysaccharide fractions in three popular blue green algae species (*AFA, Spirulina and Chlorella*) showed potent immune-stimulating activity[2]. Dr. Jensen's own team had demonstrated that consumption of AFA had rapid effects on the circulation and function of immune cells in humans. Even more definitively, it was a polysaccharide fraction that by itself induced the homing of NK cells in particular, which produced a significant transient decrease in the observed circulating NK cells. So why not measure the effect of the same polysaccharide (PS) fraction and its non-PS counterpart? That made perfect sense.

A crude polysaccharide fraction of AFA was obtained by extracting the whole blue green algae for 4 hours in 70% ethanol at 65 degrees Celsius. The ethanol extract was centrifuged and then evaporated to dryness. That yield was about 30% of the dry weight of AFA. The remaining insoluble carbohydrate - rich fraction (fraction A) was then administered to volunteers in the usual way and the results showed increased homing, leading to a **reduced** amount of both stem cells and NK cells in the peripheral blood within two hours after consumption. In contrast, consumption of the water-soluble phyco-cyanin-rich fraction of AFA did not significantly alter the number of circulating stem cells. Yet we already saw that consumption of the whole AFA led to substantial **increase** in circulating stem cells (CD34+), peaking at about two hours after intake. The conclusion must be that whatever mechanism is involved and whatever the active ingredient(s) in AFA, it was **not** the high molecular weight polysaccharides. If anything, the AFA was having an observed effect that was being even modulated downwards by the PS component. They had looked in the wrong direction that time. There was definitely something else going on. What could it be? Now they would have to hunt for the proverbial 'needle in a haystack.'

Yet, it need not be exactly so. Of all the hundreds of surface molecules that find expression on cell surfaces (and that's essentially how cells communicate), perhaps there could be just one – a special one – that would be present on a stem cell surface that might be sensitive to some active trigger or signal present in AFA. That particular surface molecule would be the one to cause stem cells to respond and be released from the bone marrow. How could the team go about finding it? Combine that low probability with a keen sense of urgency and a lack of research money and one might feel set up for disappointment and failure.

Except that there was one more strange coincidence. One of the stars of this drama, just so happens to have done her PhD thesis on a particular cell surface marker (how serendipitous is that?!). She was and still is a world expert on the subject of L-selectin. That reality turned out to be a remarkable coincidence. It weighted the odds considerably.

It is probably not surprising, but human minds always seem to gravitate to the familiar. We are programmed in fixed action patterns. We regularly confirm that every morning and every evening, and many times in- between throughout the day. But to a significant degree, we are also programmed in fixed thought patterns because in each of our worlds, common things are common. We make associations, we adhere to paradigms and we even anticipate situations and events because we are so programmed to the familiar. It's just like in art or music, in that we choose to see and hear those things that are most familiar and with which we are most comfortable.

No wonder then, that faced with the colossal challenge of finding an active ingredient in AFA and a mechanism of action for enhanced stem cell release from the bone marrow, a world expert on L-selectin is almost compelled to wonder: 'Could this AFA have anything to do with L-selectin?' That question would probably not be asked by a thousand other immunologists in the same situation. But Dr. Gitte S. Jensen is the right person, in the right place, at the right time, with the right project, to wonder about the right association and thereby set up the right assay to find the right result. Everything was just Right!

So, off to the lab they go…. and so said, so done. Dr. Jensen's team just happens to be fatefully equipped with the knowledge, the protocols, the antibodies and other reagents, the equipment … yes, everything needful to go straight for the money. They target the bull's eye and zero in. After they manage to overcome the challenges of design and execution, they eventually discover that **AFA blocks L-selectin** and ... **EUREKA!!!** For the third time. By sheer serendipity, fate appeared to have smiled on these researchers that time.

PROVING THE CASE

Here's how it happened.

This was a very sophisticated and technical challenge but from experience, Dr. Jensen and her team knew exactly what they needed to do[10]. At the risk of over simplification, we'll give just a brief outline here. They took some paramagnetic Dynabeads which were first coated with a protein G and incubated them with an L-selectin chimera protein (all commercially available products). The chimera protein was captured on the surface of the beads and subsequently bonded to it (all fairly standard procedure, like making a molecular fish hook). (Fig. 2) Then they made up a fresh extract of AFA in water (AFA-w) and added the coated beads. They captured the L-selectin binding compound from the AFA water extract which could then be separated off later.

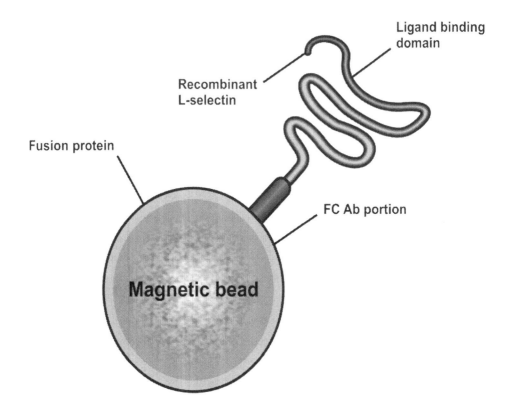

Fig. 2 AFA contains a ligand for human L-selectin

Paramagnetic Dynabeads coated with human L-selectin were incubated with a water extract of AFA. After incubation, the beads were washed and any bound material was detached and run on gel-electrophoresis. Voila ... there it was! The L-selectn blocker (ligand).

It was demonstrated to be a protein with an apparent molecular weight of about 160-180 kDa, comprised of approximately equal amounts of two smaller subunits. That's the suspect they were looking for. It's an L-selectin ligand (LSL) present in AFA (they call it the AFA-LSL). This compound is not to be confused with the much longer, water-insoluble polysaccharide in AFA, which was shown earlier to affect the activity of NK cells. This one was isolated in the water-soluble portion of AFA. They had found the culprit, now they had to prove that it was really 'guilty as charged.'

Let's just backup a minute. Recall from Chapter 2 that some cells (stem cells and immune cells in particular) express a receptor called CXCR4 that specifically recognizes the molecule released by injured tissues to attract stem cells, called stromal-cell derived factor (SDF-1). When SDF-1 binds to the CXCR4 receptor, that triggers the expression of adhesion molecules on the cell surface. This event favors retention of stem cells in the bone marrow and also adhesion to capillary walls, prior to extravasation into tissues, as in the inflammation response.

Now, there are other known L-selectin ligands, including a sulphated polysaccharide from brown algae know as fucoidan. The binding of fucoidan to L-selectin has been shown to cause cells to express the same receptor molecules known as CXCR4 on the cell surface[12]. These CXCR4 receptor molecules are actually premade inside the cell and cycle in and out in response to the trigger of L-selectin being bound in this way.

So, back to Dr. Jensen and her team who then wanted to find out if the same water soluble fraction of AFA (remember, AFA-w) would compete with fucoidan for binding L-selectin, and if it would block the externalization of CXCR4. In a nutshell, they demonstrated that it did by immuno-staining the CXCR4 expressed on the surface of different progenitor cells after exposure to AFA-w alone, to fucoidan alone and then to both. The progenitor cell types they used included bone marrow cells positive for CD34, as well as two commercially available cell lines known as KGla and K562. These two latter cell lines were specifically chosen for their differences. They are both undifferentiated, multipotent hematopoietic cell lines but only KGla is positive for CD34. The KGla cell line is also less differentiated and is more comparable to the stem cells resident in the bone marrow.

Specifically, Dr. Jensen found that the AFA-w inhibited the fucoidan-induced expression of CXCR4 only on the CD34+ cells from the bone marrow and on the KGla CD34+ cell line, but not on the CD34- (note negative) cell line K562. That would all be entirely consistent if, in fact, the L-selectin ligand did play a role in stem cell mobilization from the bone marrow. But to prove that, Dr. Jensen's team would have to move from *in vitro* experiments like those just mentioned, to real *in vivo* investigation.

To that end, they carried out a small double-blind, placebo-controlled cross over study with 12 healthy subjects. They gave either 1gm of a proprietary, patent-pending AFA preparation (commercially known as StemEnhance(R) or an equivalent placebo to these volunteers and monitored the number of CD34+ cells appearing in their peripheral blood over time. StemEnhance(R) was a unique blend of cytoplasmic and cell-wall-rich fraction of the whole AFA plant biomass, enriched about 5-fold in the content of the L-selectin ligand previously identified. They found a transient 18% increase in CD34+ stem cells (maximizing at about 1 hour after ingestion of StemEnhance(R)) relative to placebo. When volunteers failing reasonable exclusion criteria were removed from the statistical data analysis, the result was a 25% increase in CD34+ cells. To test the repeatability of the effect of consuming StemEnhance(R), 16 separate experiments were performed on a single volunteer. The average increase noted was 53%, with a median of 36% and a maximum-minimum range from 233%

at the high end, down to -4% below. All this suggests that the CD34+ cell response to the consumption of StemEnhance(R) is consistent, despite the day to day fluctuations which probably contributed to its underestimation. Interestingly, no statistically significant changes were observed for the total number of leucocytes (white blood cells) or lymphocytes, comparing StemEnhance(R) to placebo, in this entire trial.

Here's the bottom line. Dr. Jensen and her group clearly showed that **AFA contains a water-soluble active ingredient that competes for binding with L-selectin and hence reduces the expression of CXCR4 on stem cells in the bone marrow.** The earlier work done had made the team aware of how important it is to look for early results, and not miss the effect due to a bias that ' biological effects triggered by nutrients take a longer time'. The enhanced release was documented to be a rapid and transient effect that peaks in about one hour. In contrast, the known endogenous mobilizer G-CSF (granulocyte colony-stimulating factor that we met several times before) produces a much slower response that peaks only in a few days. The G-CSF is believed to break down SDF-1 by activating a series of proteolytic enzymes, thereby interfering with the SDF-1/CXCR4 axis. Its effect is much greater but its use is limited due to potentially severe side effects. Clinically it has been found that G-CSF can trigger platelet aggregation and the formation of blood clots. In rare cases, this has sometimes led to heart attack or stroke and also to a more generalized blood crisis called disseminated intravascular coagulation (DIC). Some much more common side effects that have been observed include pain (especially bone pain), gastrointestinal upset (nausea, vomiting, diarrhea), insomnia, fever, chills and night sweats. Clearly, this is unacceptable for any widespread or extended use in any attempt to enhance stem cell migration to improve health.

That leaves open the door for an alternate approach.

These astonishing results were published in the peer-reviewed journal Cardiovascular Revascularization Medicine in 2007. That important paper was coauthored by nine different scientists working in five different laboratories and bore the following descriptive title: **'Mobilization of human CD34+ CD133+ and CD34+ CD133 – stem cells in vivo by consumption of an extract from *Aphanizomenon flos-aquae* – related to modulation of CXCR4 expression by an L-selectin ligand'.** That title says it all. Nutrition and stem cells have collided to produce a new interface that has now become, **STEM CELL NUTRITION.**

Dr. Jensen and Christian Drapeau also knew that they would be on to something bigger than it appeared at that time. A second provisional application was initially filed earlier, for a Method of Use Patent, on July 19, 2005. The corresponding **Patent No: US 7, 651,690 B2** was issued to the same inventors on January 26, 2010 with the title:

'Purified Component of Blue-Green Algae and Method of Use.'

Abstract: Disclosed herein are extracts of blue-green algae, such as *Alphanizomenon flos-aque* (AFA) that are enriched for a selectin ligand, such as an L-selectin ligand. Selected ligands isolated from the blue-green algae cells are disclosed herein. Methods are described for isolating these selectin ligands. The purified selectin ligands are of use in inducing stem cell mobilization in a subject. Thus, methods for inducing stem cell isolation that include administering a therapeutically effective amount of the extract-enriched form of the selectin ligand, or an isolated selectin ligand are disclosed herein.

This patent, also assigned to Desert Lake Technologies, disclosed the process for isolating the L-selectin ligand in AFA using paramagnetic beads. They were first coated with Protein G and then a recombinant protein consisting of the extracellular portion of L-selectin, joined to a portion of a human immunoglobulin, IgG1. In this way, a new preparation derived from AFA could be made. This product would then be enriched (typically five-fold) in the active L-selectin ligand, appropriate for dietary consumption.

That brings us four-square to the leading edge of nutrition: **Stem Cell Nutrition.** This is the focus of the next chapter.

CHAPTER 6

The Leading Edge
of Nutrition

Oxidative stress is a killer. At the turn of the century, understanding of human pathophysiology had reached a stage where most professionals would probably have agreed that the biggest general cause of illness and disease was to be mediated through this process. Premature oxidation with reactive oxygen species (ROS) is a general mechanism presumed to be inherent in many degenerative illnesses and the aging process itself. It is implicated in many conditions including cancer, cardiovascular disease and inflammation (just to name a few big ones). Some dietary ingredients were proven to quench or neutralize those same lethal ROS. They were highly effective in defending the body against the ubiquitous oxidative stress. Therefore, the emphasis on supplementary antioxidants (vitamins A, C and E, glutathione precursors, CoQ10 and lycopene) could be justified at that time as the legitimate cutting edge of 'nutrition for health'.

Then came Stem Cells. They are not new. What's new is the awareness of their importance in physiology and pathology. Also new is the growth of Biotechnology that now makes it possible to begin exploiting their basic characteristics. That led to the ongoing avalanche of research and the inflated expectation of using stem cells to cure major chronic degenerative disease and even to create new ways to rebuild and restore tissues and organs of the human body. That is a daunting task with many challenges to be overcome, yet active research around the world is making slow but steady progress.

There is also something else that's new. It's the discovery just described in the previous chapter. Christian Drapeau and Dr Gitte S. Jensen demonstrated that many research reports now support their general hypothesis. The discovery of the normal renewal and healing system of the human body is slowly being recognized as a major development in physiology. Adult stem cells are naturally released from the bone marrow, then they circulate in the blood, migrate selectively into tissues, then proliferate and differentiate to replace worn out or malfunctioning cells. Furthermore, the realization that dietary intervention with certain natural products derived from substances like AFA, can enhance that renewal process in a mild but meaningful way, affords new possibilities for health and wellness. That's the new emphasis, shifting attention to the normal activity of adult stem cells and seeking to exploit the same by dietary intervention. **Such intervention defines Stem Cell (SC) Nutrition which has therefore become the new leading edge of nutrition today**.

A NEW WELLNESS STRATEGY

Why should SC Nutrition be regarded as the leading edge of nutrition today? That is a remarkable claim but it is a justifiable one. Several considerations will prove this to be true.

Before SC Nutrition was discovered, the wellness approach to health as far as nutrition was concerned, relied upon feeding the body to empower cells to remain healthy. In that way healthy cells would constitute healthy organs which would ultimately lead to a healthy body. The strategy was to provide human cells with their basic input needs. Therefore, the focus has been on vitamins and minerals, on adequate proteins, carbohydrate and essential fats. Then antioxidants came under the spotlight as leaders in the field, to counter oxidative stress inside and outside the cells. From the bench came other supporting players including fiber, supplementary enzymes, some herbal products and a couple of novel nutrient delivery systems.

But despite the input of all these essential raw materials, big questions still remained. How does the body renew itself? What happens when tissue cells malfunction or wear out and chronic degenerative processes ensue? Does the body come to rely inevitably on medical intervention with designed pharmaceutical drugs and delicate but invasive surgeries? How does the body attempt to repair or rejuvenate itself on a daily basis?

Of course, the immune system comes to mind. The body does have an elaborate and sophisticated system to protect itself. The liver functions like a detoxification plant converting harmful metabolites and foreign chemicals (including drugs) into harmless substances that get excreted. The kidneys regulate through filtration and excretion, a lot of soluble waste products and do so in a most efficient manner. Then of course, at the cellular level, the body has an integrated system of cells that generally circulate as a defense force. They target any type of harmful enemy that invades, including pathogens like bacteria, viruses and protozoa. Some cells carry out surveillance maneuvers and detect the enemy. Others tag the enemy and prepare it for destruction, by whatever means necessary, while others come in for the kill and still others are left for mop- up operations. Some smart cells keep a record (and help keep a mean score) in anticipation of any repeat attack. It is biological war at a personal level.

That's just the beginning, because there's so much more to the immune system. Research in this area has led to major developments in medicine such as vaccines that have saved millions of lives, blood transfusion and organ transplant to restore function when failure was inevitable, or the advances made in the diagnosis and management of autoimmune diseases – just to name a few.

However, it is hard to believe that until recently, we had overlooked the natural repair and renewal system that operates continuously in both health and disease. It took a long time to appreciate the true nature of stem cells, but once researchers got a handle on these pluripotent 'possibilities', it seemed that the area of regenerative medicine could not be very far away. The reports in the media especially, and the prospects for real breakthroughs began to sound more like fiction than science. And in that frenzy, what now seems so obvious and so important went under the radar screen. That was until Christian Drapeau and Dr. Gitte Jensen put it together in their now famous hypothesis that is being increasingly validated by research reports coming out of many centers.

Adult stem cells from the bone marrow have been shown to support the health of most systems in the human body. These include the health of the central nervous system,[1] the cardiovascular system,[2] and the functions of the liver,[3] kidney,[4] pancreas,[5] lung,[6] skin[7] and bone.[8] And that's not all. This is the normal renewal system taking place in every body, every day. Recall the mantra: **Everybody has stem cells; everybody uses stem cells; everybody uses stem cells everyday; stem cells work … and they work every time.**

This is a crucial advance in our understanding of how the body maintains and renews itself. The focus is not on the invading enemy. It is on local defense through local maintenance. Every day of our lives stem cells emerge from our bone marrow and circulate in the peripheral blood, migrating into tissues that need assistance. Tissues wear out, they are sometimes attacked, or they malfunction. Cells deteriorate and die. Therefore there is constant need for maintenance and repair, for renewal and healing on the local home front. Stem cells go a long way in supporting that internal effort. In fact, so much so that we now understand that the number of stem cells circulating in the blood stream is indeed a determining factor for overall health. Why? If more stem cells circulate, then more stem cells are available for this daily natural process of repair throughout the body and that can only lead to better health.

But as a strategy for wellness, the discovery of that renewal process is only the first half of the complete equation. The second half is just as significant and just as surprising in its apparent simplicity. The discovery that a dietary intervention that we have chosen to call **Stem Cell Nutrition** (therefore, that forms the title of this book - just in case) presents a new wellness strategy from a fundamental point of view. In a nutshell, we can now move - by simple ingestion of natural products - from the particular cells of the body to the general body itself, from the local to the total. We shift focus from protecting cells to providing replacement cells. In this way we pivot from degradation to restoration. Tissue maintenance involves more than cellular sustenance, it requires regular renewal and repair with new tissue cells that necessarily derive from the bone marrow.

Let's express that another way. Typically, dietary supplementation, as best exemplified by multivitamin preparations, has been designed to supply nourishment to old cells. These are the typical cells of organ and tissues that are exposed to daily insults of every kind and struggle to survive. They get beat up, degraded, derailed from within and finally stagger at the count until in turn, they begin to die off. In a sense the multivitamin supplements help those cells to put up a good fight, but they really only delay the inevitable.

In contrast, SC Nutrition is designed to support the natural release of 'master' cells. These are the fresh, vibrant and versatile cellular marines that can transform themselves into healthy new recruit cells. That process of recruitment restores and refreshes tissues on the frontlines in a most healthful way that the body can now celebrate in optimum wellness. That principally puts SC Nutrition at the leading edge of nutrition.

Wellness advocates have always believed in the intrinsic ability of the human body to heal itself. The mantra was: 'give the body the tools and it would do the job.' But we never quite knew how - until now. The natural renewal process involving stem cells from the bone marrow provides a major key. Stem Cell Nutrition now opens the door. It's a door to better health and wellness. More stem cells are released from the bone marrow and go on their mission of renewal and restoration, getting their job done with excellence and efficiency in a way that only such pluripotent stem cells can. The net results are nothing less than better health, reduced illness, enhanced performance and the vitality and vigor that characterizes such an experience of optimized wellness. This can become an unassailable strategy - a strategy based on SC Nutrition – it is nutrition at the leading edge.

In the remainder of this chapter we want to consider three basic questions that arise about this new strategy:

(i)   What other possible natural products besides a proprietary AFA concentrate can or does enhance stem cell release from the bone marrow?

(ii) What other ways might exist for products like these to influence stem cell physiology other than by just enhancing the release from the bone marrow? And finally,

(iii) What other possible health benefits may be derived from the superstar of our show, AFA?

OTHER STEM CELL ENHANCERS

In response to the first question that was just raised, it would be really surprising if the sulfated glycans found in the blue green algae AFA, were the only naturally occurring edible stem cell enhancers. Surely there must be others. It would be further surprising if it turned out that blocking the crucial L-selectin was the only mechanism by which the release of stem cells from the bone marrow could be enhanced. It is not uncommon in nature to find that many crucial biological processes have alternate routes as if, just in case, assurance is made doubly sure.

During the past few years, a few other natural substances have also been shown to enhance stem cell release from the bone marrow. In fact, we have already met one of these in Chapter 2, where we referred to another L-selectin blocker, known generally as fucoidan.

Fucoidan

Fucoidans are really a class of sulfated polysaccharides found mainly in various species of brown algae and seaweed such as *mozuku, wakame, kombu, hijiki and bladdewrack*. Variant forms of fucoidan have also been found in animal species like the sea cucumber. The most common source of experimental fucoidan in the published literature is derived from *Fucus vesiculosis* which is a common harvest crop of a northern hemisphere kelp. This fucoidan, like all primary fucoidan extracts is heterodisperse and contains a high percentage of *fucose*. On the other hand, some of the popular Asian seaweeds like *Undaria pinnatifida* contain a different sugar, *galactose*.

For centuries these fucoidan-containing seaweeds have been prized in Asian cultures for their dietary and medicinal properties. Fucoidan itself has been recognized for several decades as having a key role in the biology of the seaweed and its activity has been examined in research laboratories around the world (in Australia, Japan, Korea, Russia, China as well as Europe and the Americas). The intensity of fucoidan effects on human physiology and other biological activities varies quite a lot. It depends on the particular species, molecular weight (average is about 20,000 Da), composition, structure and the route of administration (intravenous or oral). The biological effects are quite interesting and a number of pharmaceutical companies have pursued the possibilities, although these companies have generally preferred smaller, well defined molecules that can be more readily exploited as drugs.

However, carefully controlled sources of seaweed as well as modern extraction and characterization methods are now being used commercially to produce well defined fucoidan derivatives of high quality. For example, Marinova, a progressive Australian biotechnology company, has been developing innovative medical and nutritional applications from marine plants. Their R&D has been focused on fucoidans derived from *Undaria pinnatifida* and they have a modern extraction facility in Cambridge, Tasmania. They use a water-based patented process to isolate high-purity, organic fucoidan extracts using a variety of seaweeds from Tasmania, Nova Scotia, Patagonia and the Pacific Islands.

Published research on the physiological effects of fucoidan has demonstrated that it does have significant anti- inflammatory activity. As such, it inhibits selectins,[9] complement[10] and some enzymes.[11] *Selectins* are cell surface receptors on white blood cells that make them 'sticky', allowing them to 'roll' on an organ's endothelial surface and enter that tissue space. Blocking the selectin, reduces the adhesion and 'rolling', thereby reducing inflammation on whole organs like the heart, kidneys, or liver. *Complement* is a cascade system of about 30 enzymes (proteins) in the blood serum that helps to regulate immunity and limit bleeding. Fucoidan can inhibit both the formation and binding of different complement factors. It can also inhibit several *enzymes* that cause tissue breakdown when inflammation does occur.

There are still other physiological effects of fucoidan. It is known to reduce pain in osteoarthritis[12], even though the mechanism of action is still somewhat unclear. Techniques have been developed using fucoidan as an ingredient in a loaded film format that inhibits the number of post surgical adhesions in a rabbit model by up to 90%, without toxicity[13]. Probably acting as a selectin blocker, post-ischemic inflammation is reduced and the subsequent fibrotic reaction contained. Similarly, after toxic or pathogenic insults to the liver, fibrosis often sets in and liver function is compromised. Fucoidan has been demonstrated to be a highly effective inhibitor of this type of fibrosis.[14] It has also been known to have anti-viral activity[15] not by killing viruses, but by first reducing their entry into cells (by blocking receptors) and then interfering with their replication.

Despite all those other physiological effects of fucoidan, the main effect that is of interest here is that of mobilizing stem cells. Fucoidan is known to increase the release of stem cells from the bone marrow and into the bloodstream, when administered intravenously or orally[16]. The fucoidan from *Fucus vesiculosis* (rich in fucose) has been known to do this in baboons and mice. The mechanism seems to involve both the inhibition of selectin binding as well as the ability of fucoidan to bind to stromal cell-derived factor-1 (SDF-1/CXCL12)[17]. However, when that same fucoidan derivative was injected intra-peritoneally into rats after serious damage to their livers, the binding of fucoidan to SDF-1 was, rather surprisingly, found to block liver regeneration in this animal model.[18]

In a more definitive clinical study in this area, Irhimeh and co-workers at the University of Tasmania in Australia administered a specific concentration of fucoidan from *Undaria pinnatifida* orally to human volunteers in a clinical trial[16]. They found that ingestion of fucoidan led to a significant increase in the number of both CD 34+ cells in peripheral blood and the levels of SDF-1, all within days. At the same time, the proportion of the hematopoietic progenitor cells that expressed the CXCR4 receptors was also increased. This all correlates with earlier *in vitro* and *animal* studies that showed fucoidan mobilizes stem cells.

It is also reassuring to know that fucoidan derived from all species of brown algae have shown no signs of toxicity *in vitro* or *in vivo*. Recent toxicology reports prove that fucoidan from *Undaria pinnatifida* and *Laminaria japonica* was safe in animal models at very high levels of ingestion[19]. Human clinical studies using oral consumption at doses of 1 gram per day for up to three months (chronic use), or 3 grams per day for 12 days (acute use), also showed no signs of toxicity.[16] However, it is noteworthy that fucoidan can influence coagulation (in a reversible way) at higher doses[20] and should therefore be cautiously restricted whenever blood homeostasis is an issue.

The net conclusion from all this research on fucoidan is that, in addition to whatever other benefits may be derived, oral intake of a good source such as the specific concentration of *Undaria pinnatifida* used in clinical trials, effectively enhances stem cell release in its own right and can therefore be a useful addition to SC Nutrition. Moreover, compared to AFA extract, the response to fucoidan was delayed but also more prolonged. Therefore, a combination of both stem cell enhancers should lead to an early response yes, but also to one that is more prolonged. This does indeed prove to be the case.

Polygonum Multiflorum

Another natural product that has been shown to be an effective stem cell enhancer is an ancient Chinese herb commonly known as *fo-ti* or *Foti*. The plant is native to China but is also found in Japan and

Taiwan. The root is the medicinally active part and it is traditionally used as a tonic for a variety of common symptoms and conditions.

The story behind *Foti* is interesting in its own way. In Chinese medicine there is the concept of *Chi*, which is fairly well known even here in the West. It refers generally to the 'energy' in the body that ebbs and flows, waxes and wanes, subject to definitive factors which can be manipulated (to advantage),in various ways, leading to overall health and wellness as a result.

There is another concept that also relates to energy, but in a different modality. It is called the *Jing* which is also quite well known in modern Chinese medicine. But in the ancient or more traditional use, the concept was somewhat different than it is today. First, there was the so-called 'primordial *Jing*' that is present at conception and leads to development of the human body. But there is also another *Jing* which is present after birth. This second 'residual *Jing*,' plays a very important role throughout life in healing and repair, in regeneration and rejuvenation. These complementary concepts seem to almost parallel the known role of embryonic stem cells and *adult* stem cells, so it would not be an unfair extrapolation to try to relate this ancient 'Jing philosophy' to the modern understanding of stem cells.

What that simple hypothesis did was to prompt an enquiry into what natural products were associated, at least in ancient Chinese Medicine with the promotion and enhancement of the *Jing* in the body. That might provide a clue to possibly help identify alternative natural products that could enhance stem cell release too. It was a small guiding light in the dim twilight (if not total darkness) that pervaded research minds looking for other possible stem cell enhancers. The fact is that there were only a few candidates from the contemporary Chinese medicine repertoire that were known to be outstanding supporters of *Jing*, and therefore really worthy of serious consideration in this regard. This narrowed the field considerably.

After testing a number of these natural products, only one proved to be truly effective in enhancing stem cell release in a small human trial. That was *Foti*, or more technically, *Polygonum multiflorum*. An extract of this fine herb that has a long history of use to support health and rejuvenation, was documented to support the release of stem cells from the bone marrow. The effect was smaller, compared to AFA and fucoidan, but it was there.

This *Foti* plant has been associated with legends that are only referred to here for their anecdotal interest. Another name for *Foti* is *He Shon Wu* which translates as a 'black- haired' Mr. He. This is in reference to an old villager (a Mr. He) who took *Foti* and restored his black hair, youthful appearance and vitality. Legend has it that he lived to be 130 years of age, after his father and grandfather had both lived to a ripe old age themselves. The story goes on to tell that the grandfather was impotent to age 58 and took to drinking wine. One evening, he returned home drunk and fell asleep in the field outside his home. When he awoke, he noticed a couple of climbing plants at his side that twisted around each other. He perceived a message of love and sexuality coming from these plants. After fruitless inquiries about the plants in the village, he was eventually told by a jester living nearby that they might contain a divine drug that could work wonders. Mr. He found a way to pulverize the root of the plant and consumed the powder with his wine. It did work wonders. The plant turned out to be young shoots of real Foti. He later married a widow, fathered 9 children and lived, as the story goes, to 160 years of age. So goes the legend - for what it is worth.

But there is clearly more to *Foti* than mere legend. Some scientific studies have actually been done that at least suggest that *Foti* extract can improve the cardiovascular system, enhance immune functions, slow the degeneration of endocrine glands, increase antioxidant activity and limit lipid peroxidation.[21] In Chinese medicine, it does have that anti-aging association, among many other applications.

Unfortunately, in higher doses *Foti* has been shown to sometimes have significant side effects.[22] It has been known to cause gastrointestinal upset, skin rash (hypersensitivity), potassium deficiency with muscle weakness, numbness and even hallucinations. In the most extreme cases, hepatitis has been observed, such that this plant is probably contraindicated for patients with liver disease. In the interest of caution, it is also probably wise to avoid during pregnancy and breast feeding.

Having said all that, it is wise to maintain perspective. Millions of people have used *Foti* for centuries and there have hardly been any reports of severe adverse effects with normal use. Any minimal usage as a synergistic ingredient in a formula designed to enhance stem cell release should be no reason for concern or anxiety in terms of any significant side effects.

SYNERGY

The practical concept of 'synergy' is well recognized. It is often found in reality that with respect to collective effect involving different components, 'the total is more than the sum of the parts'. The simple realization is that sometimes when you put things together, you observe or derive a benefit that is more than you would expect from mere addition of the individual contributions. Such is a symphony. Each musician plays a singular part of the composition, but the audience witnessing the full concert of sound knows nothing of the distinct separate parts played by each instrument. It is an experience that is extracted as a production by the conductor as he or she directs. That's the expression of synergy in music. The same may be said of any professional team sport. The individual players may be stars in their own right, possessing an abundance of talent and skills that command astronomical salaries. But the performance of any winning team is determined in the final analysis by the cooperation and coordination of all the players that combine to execute miraculous precision and finesse that is a beauty to behold as they claim victory over the opposing team. That's the expression of synergy in team sport.

So it is also with SC Nutrition. The enhancement of stem cell release from the bone marrow is optimized in a dramatic way by combining the effect of different stem cell enhancers to derive a good early response that is sustained over several hours. With AFA extract alone, there was observed in clinical study, an increase of 20 – 30 percent in circulating stem cells. The effect peaked after about 60 minutes and then slowly returned to baseline levels. With *Undaria pinnatifida*, there was a slower increase in the number of stem cells in circulation, but the effect lasted much longer. The total increase in the number of stem cells released for an equivalent amount of the enhancer was about 50 percent more for Undaria than for AFA. For *Polygonum multiflorum*, the effect was comparable to AFA, peaking at about 60 minutes, but smaller in its overall effect. When all three of these components are blended or combined, a significantly stronger response was realized and the effect lasted much longer. Fig. 3 illustrates this 'synergy', extending the elevated levels of stem cells in the peripheral blood for several hours. That's the expression of synergy in SC Nutrition.

Again, it is worth emphasizing that this is a powerful effect of increasing the number of circulating adult stem cells, which we now know is highly indicative of advantages to health and wellbeing. It is an appropriate 'marker' that relates to the overall health risk of an individual.[7] With more stem cells in the bloodstream, one can infer a lower risk of developing degenerative disease. That's a principal objective of the 'wellness' approach. Perhaps even more important is the emphasis here that through SC Nutrition, one can conveniently increase this adult stem cell population to promote optimum health.

That's clearly on the leading edge of nutrition today.

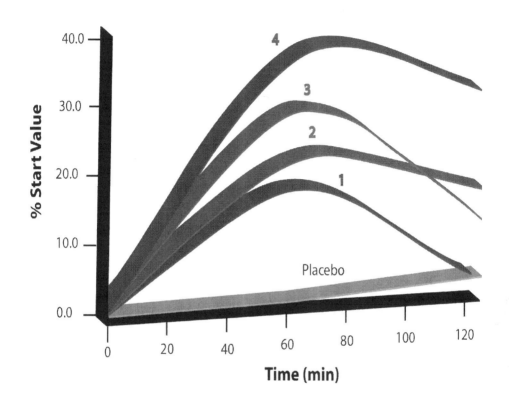

Fig3. Synergy of Enhanced Stem Cell Release.

The effect on release of stem cells from the bone marrow is shown here, after human consumption of AFA(1), Polygonum multiflorum extract(2) , Undaria pinnatifida(3) and a specific combination of all three(4).

RELEASE, CIRCULATE, MIGRATE

Now we come to the second question that was raised earlier. What other ways might exist for natural dietary products like those we have been considering, to influence stem cell physiology other than by just enhancing stem cell release from the bone marrow?

We have already discussed in some detail the normal activity of stem cells. That was much earlier in Chapter Two. Clearly, the physiology of these pluripotent lifesavers goes well beyond just their release from the bone marrow. We also described earlier a six-step process that eventually leads to the normal renewal and healing activity that stem cells execute continuously. However, from a nutritional point of view there are three most important areas of support that can and should be addressed specifically.

We have already gone into much detail regarding the effect of natural stem cell enhancers that focused on the **release** step in the overall process. That's the important first step. Understanding this should lead the reader to have a high regard for the benefits to be derived from certain clinically-studied concentrations of *Aphanizomenon flos aquae* (AFA), *Undaria pinnatifida (fucoidan)*, and *Polygonum multiforum (Foti)* which act in concert to produce a good early and yet sustained effect of increasing the number of circulating stem cells released from the bone marrow. What a great start for SC Nutrition! **Supplementation with such a blend is perhaps the single most important thing that one can do routinely to optimize stem cell physiology.**

However, after the stem cells are released from the bone marrow, they must **circulate** in the blood to get to the 'presumed tissues in need'. The bloodstream is the body's superhighway. It carries all the traffic, with important nutrients and vital oxygen, hormones, immune cells, platelets for clotting, drugs (when indicated), some waste products (en route to the liver for detoxification or to the kidneys for elimination) and even more. That 'more' we now understand, includes the very important stem cells – the pluripotent lifesavers – destined to fulfill a mission of support. This mission involves the maintenance and renewal of worn-out or malfunctioning cells that put tissues at risk.

The all important blood circulation tapers down from the superhighway into increasingly smaller pathways, until the cells can travel only in single file. This dynamic system can be impaired for many reasons. SC Nutrition would seek to maintain good effective blood flow and that involves the cardiovascular system in general. That calls for a healthy heart (*cardio-*) and clean, smooth healthy vessels (*-vascular*). In that regard, diets that are low in fat, LDL cholesterol and salt, as well as high in fiber, go a long way to aid SC Nutrition in the most general sense. This of course, is to be complemented with a lifestyle that favors heart health. That includes saying No! to smoking, managing diabetes where present, maintaining blood pressure to control any essential hypertension, getting moderate exercise and effectively managing stress.

In a more particular way, significant damage to the cardiovascular system is known to develop as a consequence of 'oxidative stress', which of course gave rise to the 'antioxidant revolution' we referred to in Chapter 4. This type of premature or inappropriate cellular oxidation leads to inflammation which impedes the normal cardiovascular physiology in significant ways. For example, in a review of 'Oxidative Stress, Inflammation and Diabetic Complications' in a classic textbook on Diabetes Mellitus, the authors concluded with this statement: *"Significant evidence from experimental, animal and human studies supports the role of oxidative stress and inflammation in the development of diabetic microvascular and macrovascular complications"*[23]. We would expect these effects even in normal individuals to potentially obstruct the effective transport or flow of stem cells to the needy tissues. Therefore, antioxidants could in effect help to minimize this oxidative inhibition.

Nutritionally, antioxidants in the diet have been shown to counter the effects of oxidative stress and reduce inflammation, thereby supporting blood flow and the microvasculature (tiny capillaries etc.) in particular[24]. Some of the best antioxidant botanicals include *Indian Gooseberry* (amla) which is a potent super-fruit with strong antioxidant benefits and clinically shown to support cardiovascular circulation. *Black Currant* is a different berry, native to northern Europe and Asia, with very high antioxidant content, including vitamin C as well. It too supports stem cell function. Similarly, there is *mangosteen* an extraordinary fruit originally from Southeast Asia that is well known for its antioxidant properties. So also is *cat's claw* the 'sacred herb of the rainforest'. This is a tropical vine from the jungles of the Amazonian Basin, which does have potent antioxidant effect. We could also mention other sources like *vitis vinifera* (grape) seeds and pomace which may contain up to 80 percent polyphenols (known to be rich antioxidants), as well as the more common *citrus* fruits rich in bioflavonoids like hesperidin. There are many more.

Still on the subject of stem cells in the microcirculation, a further consideration would be the tendency sometimes for blood to form very small clots. This could be due to an excess of fibrin (a clotting factor) that could build up in these very tiny blood vessels. Some active fibrinolytic enzymes have been clinically shown to digest excess fibrin to help clear the pathway of the circulatory system[25,26]. This too could form part of any package of natural products designed to improve the flo' of blood carrying stem cells to their destination of renewal and repair. Obviously, patients with bleeding disorders or those on anti-coagulant medications should consult their healthcare practitioners before engaging in this type of intervention.

One more strategy to help maintain adequate flow where it really matters is the principle of detoxification. This is a concept not wide-ly exploited in Western allopathic medicine except in the narrow area of toxicology. The latter relates more to exogenous poisons and overindulgence in some form (like in drug abuse, metal ingestion, childhood experimentation, etc.) But that's not so in the practice of Eastern traditional or Western complementary medicine. The con-cept there relates more to a different paradigm in which, over time unwanted 'toxins' (both exogenous and endogenous) accumulate in the bloodstream and these need to be removed. Several possible mechanisms for this have been suggested. Toxins could be prepared for capture, filtration and elimination via the liver and/or kidneys. Alternatively, one might increase any tendency to 'sweat' such 'tox-ins' off, through the pores of the skin. Whatever the case may be, there is the general appreciation that in alternative/complementary medicine practice, the blood circulation in particular (and the body in general), benefits from natural detoxifying effects of specific agents. One example might be a product like *curcumin* from the turmeric plant. *Curcumin* has been used for centuries, in Asia for example, to help 'purify the blood' and 'detoxify the body'. Similar properties can be ascribed to the mineral '*Silicate*', known for a long time as a strong antioxidant and detoxifying agent.

Again, when it comes to supporting blood flo', synergy is the key. The combined benefits of different ingredients – nutritional antioxi-dants and anti-inflammatory agents, plus fibrinolytic enzymes and detoxifying agents – can prove to be more than the sum of the indi-vidual contributions. But the important goal remains - optimizing blood flow to the finest capillaries in every single tissue of the body, to simply get the job done. It's so important to get those stem cells where they belong, executing their mission of maintenance and heal-ing at the tissue points of need.

So does this all add up? Can SC Nutrition support the microcircula-tion? The proven answer is 'Yes!' But is there any evidence that this is indeed the case?

There is only one way to effectively estimate blood circulation through tiny capillaries, and that is by measuring the diffusion of oxygen through the skin. More oxygen released by the skin means more oxygen in the underlying capillaries, which in turn means better circulation of blood. The combined effect of a proprietary blend of all the types of ingredients mentioned above was shown (by this oxygen diffusion method) to improve capillary circulation within 30 minutes of consumption. Laboratory indicators of fibrin levels and oxidative stress in the blood were also reduced at the same time[27].

That brings us to the final step where SC Nutrition can make a further difference. When stem cells arrive in the tissues that need support, they must leave the microcirculation and **migrate** to the tissue and to the exact locus of need.

Naturally, as we go further into the renewal process where stem cells are now migrating from the tiny microvasculature, one cell at a time into the surrounding tissue, it becomes less obvious how SC Nutrition can effectively influence the outcome. It is therefore not surprising that researchers have relied on a more generalized approach. They have identified a number of traditional natural substances that were good candidates for this role and tested them in the laboratory for any evidence of support for the migration of adult stem cells. Of those natural products tested, the top four performers have been identified :

Goji fruit extract – This is derived from the bright orange-red 'superfruit', and contains polysaccharides that have been shown to function as powerful antioxidants in aged mice.

Ganoderma lucidum – This is a mushroom that grows on some hardwoods and has been used as a herbal remedy in traditional Asian medicines. This particular species contains a number of bioactive compounds including enzymes that digest cellulose, lignin and xylan. It is being investigated for a variety of therapeutic effects including anti- cancer, immuno-regulatory, antioxidant and more.

Cherdaria cladosiphan– This is a species of brown algae found in the ocean. As a salt-water plant, it contains fucoidan, the important stem cell enhancer. In effect, fucoidan seems to enhance not only the release of stem cells from the bone marrow in one species, but also their migration into tissues in another.

Colostrum: Bovine colostrum is a form of 'early milk' produced by the mammary glands of cows in late pregnancy and just after birth. This popular animal product and its derivatives have been promoted by alternative or complementary health practitioners for a long time. As a health product it is generally safe for human consumption and is known to have a variety of bioactive ingredients that have been investigated for possible physiological benefit.

All four of these natural ingredients have been clinically shown to support the migration of adult stem cells out of the blood and into tissue where they are needed. But again, how can we be sure?

Recall from Chapter 2, that in the normal activity of stem cells, activation of the L-selectin on the stem cell surface causes more expression of CXCR4 receptors. These receptors then bind to the SDF-1 secreted by bone marrow or by any injured tissue. In the bone marrow, **blocking** of L-selectin favors release of the stem cells. Here in the tissue, the opposite is the case. The **activation** of L-selectin leads to attraction and attachment of the stem cells to the injured tissue. In other words, that promotes migration into the tissue.

Now then, in the case of all four natural ingredients just mentioned above, when tested for effects on stem cells, the results prove that they all exhibit agonist tendencies - they activate the L-selectin and increase CXCR4 expression[27]. So although there is no known way to verify the actual migration step, we know that the relevant favourable factors are promoted by these natural ingredients. That`s as much as we know and as much as we can say for sure, for now. As they contribute to this third stage (in the simplified triad: release, circulate and migrate), they make obvious their role in the overall strategy of SC Nutrition.

Yet there is still more good news. The benefits of certain SC Nutrition substances go even beyond the natural renewal system. There are other positive healthful effects.

OTHER BENEFITS OF AFA

We come now to the third and final question we asked earlier. What other possible health benefits may be derived from the superstar of our show – AFA? The answer proves to be quite impressive.

It began during the unscheduled meeting at the airport referred to in the previous chapter. That was when Christian Drapeau first proposed to Howard Newman that he wanted to rebrand AFA and expand the market for this remarkable blue green algae that was being credited via anecdotal reports for different health benefits associated with its consumption. Then as they teamed up with Dr. Gitte Jensen and started their laboratory work on the physiological effects of different AFA fractions, they began to discover some of the basic reasons why so many consumers were excited about the health improvements they were experiencing.

But that's never really surprising with edible natural products. Food comes in packaged form and not as isolated chemicals. In each package there are varieties of nutrients that generally have a range of physiological activity in the body. When consumed and assimilated, they each go about their mission, delivering all the benefits they were designed to provide. All food products tend to do that normally, without any human direction or script. *Aphanizomenon flos aquae* is therefore no exception. It does deliver other benefits besides the enhancement of stem cell release from the bone marrow. Three of these are of particular interest so we choose to include them here. They pertain to changes in mood, immune modulation and anti-oxidation/inflammation effects.

Elevated Mood

There is no doubt that over the past two decades at least, some consumers of AFA have reported quite frequently that they observed a distinct elevation of mood, improved mental alertness and concentration, plus a general heightened feeling of well being after consuming these products. Considering the characterized ingredients of AFA, there is only one immediate suspect that is known to have this kind of biological effect. That is the monoamine alkaloid chemically identified as phenylethylamine (PEA).

The anecdotal psychological benefits from consuming AFA do correlate with the fact that the PEA is well known for its ability to release noradrenalin[28] and dopamine[29]. Dopamine is a neurotransmitter hormone in the central nervous system that has a clear role in the feeling of wellbeing, while noradrenalin is a stimulant hormone that increases heart rate, blood pressure and general blood flow. Therefore when such hormones are increased there is an improvement in mood as well as exercise performance (through increased delivery of blood with nutrients to the tissues).

However, as attractive as such an explanation may be, there is the biochemical caveat that when PEA is ingested by mouth and absorbed, there is rapid metabolism in its first-pass through the liver, so that its half life is around 5 to 10 minutes[30]. The well known enzyme (from pharmacology) referred to as monoamine oxidase (MAO) rapidly converts PEA into phenylacetic acid, which would tend to prevent significant concentrations from reaching the brain- all other things being equal.

But, given the strength of the unsolicited anecdotal reports over time, 'all other things may not be equal'. We do know that PEA is naturally occurring in the brain. Just as exercise produces more endorphins which are endogenous opioids, the body also naturally makes PEA[31]. Nature was first and then came pharmacology, much, much later. In any case, PEA is synthesized in the body by enzymatic decarboxylation of the amino acid, phenylalanine. This same amino acid is itself found in many foods such as meat, fish, eggs, milk and nuts- to name a few. We also know that PEA acts as a neuro-modulator or -transmitter in the central nervous system[32]. Abnormally low levels of PEA have been demonstrated in patients with depression[33] and attention deficit and/or hyperactivity disorder (ADHD)[34]. Studies have shown that PEA can relieve symptoms of depression, even in some patients who were unresponsive to other more standard treatments[35,36]. The mechanism of action could probably be related to the stimulation of dopamine release, and what is significantly interesting about that is the fact that PEA improves mood without producing any associated tolerance or withdrawal.

Apart from its natural occurrence in AFA, PEA has made its way into other dietary supplement formulas. Such products have sometimes been promoted as weight loss supplements because when PEA apparently improves mood, it can potentially also reduce appetite. Some go further to suggest that when PEA stimulates noradrenalin and delays its reuptake, this favors increased lipolysis (fat breakdown). Clearly, this type of activity would be unrelated to any effects resulting from the small amounts of PEA consumed as a natural ingredient in AFA.

That last statement could also be underlined with respect to any possible side effects that PEA may cause under extreme conditions. They do not relate to SC Nutrition in any way. But on a positive note, because PEA occurs naturally in AFA, and is therefore also included as one ingredient in an organic package comprised of the necessary support players, the synergy of all the AFA components acting in concert cannot be underestimated. All things may indeed not be equal when nature is compared to pharmacology.

Immune Modulation

One of the earliest studies done at McGill by Dr. Jensen and her research group when they first turned their attention to AFA, was to examine the short term effects of consuming relatively moderate amounts (1.5 grams) of the microalgae on the immune system. Based on the many case reports of immunological effects of consuming AFA itself, and also given the documented immuno-modulatory antiviral and antibacterial properties of AFA's cousin, Spirulina, this seemed to be a promising area for basic research.

They therefore did a cross-over, placebo controlled, randomized, double blind trial with 21 volunteers, including 5 long term AFA consumers[37]. They demonstrated that consuming small moderate amounts of AFA resulted in rapid changes in immune cell trafficking. They observed two hours after AFA consumption, a generalized mobilization of lymphocytes and monocytes, but not polymorph nucleated cells. In addition, the relative proportions and absolute numbers of natural killer cells (NK) were reduced at the same time. There was also a mild but significant reduction in phagocytic activity (the ability to snatch up other cells, usually to destroy them) for the polymorphs. However, when freshly purified lymphocytes were exposed to AFA extract *in vitro* , no direct activation was induced.

One might suspect a direct effect of AFA, whereby bioactive ingredient molecules could be absorbed into the blood, transported to the bone marrow and spleen, and there cause cellular changes leading to the release of immune cells. However, a more plausible model for explaining all the observations was that immune or neuro-active substances in AFA lead to triggering of a gut-to-brain communication via the abdominal vagus nerve. That would trigger brain-to-lymphoid signals, including the rapid release of chemokines. This was consistent with the observation that the recirculation of lymphocytes was stronger in long-term AFA consumers. That would also suggest a CNS-conditioning to preferentially recognize the stimulation triggered by AFA in previously exposed subjects. At the same time, there was no evidence of direct activation of any component of the immune system, or even a general activation of the immune system as a whole. That could otherwise prove deleterious in different circumstances. But the increased trafficking of selective immune cells could translate into better surveillance, patrolling for microbial invaders as well as virus-infected or transformed cells.

In a follow up study to this trial a few years later, Dr. Jensen and colleagues identified a particular extract from AFA that was able to directly activate NK cells *in vitro* and modulate their chemokine receptor profile[38]. The NK cells play a key role in immune surveillance. They provide primary defense that we alluded to earlier, against viral infections and cancer, partly because they have the ability to destroy virally infected cells and some tumor cells without prior sensitization. They also contribute to anti-bacterial defense, which does require prior phagocytosis (engulfing) by macrophage cells. They also help maintain a healthy composition of flora in the intestinal tract.

In light of all that, any effect of AFA on stimulating NK activity offers interesting possibilities for dietary immune modulation via NK cells. We already noted that AFA consumption resulted in a transient reduction in peripheral blood NK cells in the previous randomized double blind trial. The *in vitro* study showed clearly an induction of CD69 expression on the NK cells, but even more importantly, a down regulation of the CXCR4 receptor. You may recall that latter one as the receptor that specifically recognizes the stromal cell-derived factor-1 (SDF-1) which plays a key role in recruiting NK cells into the bone marrow environment. But it appears that the NK cells become more sensitive to other chemotactic signals, thereby increasing the homing to tissues other than bone marrow as part of immune surveillance. This may occur first in the lymphoid tissue of the intestines and afterwards trigger a cascade of other immune events.

The characterization of the active ingredients in this case appears to show that smaller soluble peptides are also involved rather than the much larger polysaccharides in other fractions of AFA known to also have immune-modulatory effects. These larger water-soluble polysaccharides (also related to similar derivatives from its 'cousins': Spirulina and Chlorella) have been reported to primarily activate macrophages. Finally, to put this in perspective, these polysaccharides are between 100 – 1000 times more active for *in vitro* monocyte activation than polysaccharide preparations that have been used clinically for cancer immunotherapy.[39]

Anti-oxidation, Anti-inflammation

The third major additional benefit to be derived from the consumption of AFA, relates to the action of one of the major pigment constituents that it contains. This pigment called phycocyanin (Pc) helps to impart the characteristic color to the blue green algae (cyanobacteria) that includes AFA and its 'related cousin', Spirulina. The perceived benefit of both these microalgae have been celebrated for a long time, due in part to their antioxidant and anti-inflammatory properties, now known to be associated with the Pc which they contain.

Phycocyanin derives its name from the Greek *phyco* for algae and the English *cyan* which is a shade of blue-green (aqua). Cyan has its root in Greek *kyanos* which really is a dark blue color. It is a pigment protein complex comprised of two dissimilar alpha- and beta- protein subunits of larger molecular weights (17,000 and 19,500 Da respectively). These subunits contain linear tetrapyrrole chromophores covalently attached. Phycocyanin is an accessory pigment to chlorophyll, the all important green pigment in plants that converts carbon dioxide into carbohydrates and oxygen by photosynthesis.

Phycocyanin can be fairly easily separated from the microalgae, and its properties have been studied quite extensively *in vitro*. Such studies have clearly shown by a variety of experimental methods, that it is an efficient scavenger of oxygen free radicals and that it also reacts with other oxidizing species of pathological relevance such as HOCl and ONOO (nitrate) anion.

As we mentioned at the beginning of this chapter, there are several diseases that are accompanied (or even caused) by oxidative stress. These are typically characterized by the excessive formation of ROS that cannot be effectively counteracted by the inherent antioxidant defense system of the organism (including humans). Hence the application of exogenous antioxidants, either natural or less desirably synthetic, has been of therapeutic relevance[40].

The list of ROS that have been shown to be scavenged by phycocyanin in vitro is rather lengthy. Just a few examples should suffice.

- Alkoxyl (RO) and hydroxyl (HO) radicals were demonstrated to be quenched by phycocyanin using a chemiluminescense assay[41].

- Phycocyanin can be bleached by peroxyl radicals derived from thermolysis of a common initiator, AAPH. The ability of other antioxidant substances to protect Pc against this effect has even been proposed as a methodology to evaluate the oxygen radical absorbing capacity (ORAC) of such substances[42].

-Lipid peroxidation by ROS is known to cause damage and destruction of cell membranes. Pc significantly inhibits the increase of lipid peroxides in rat liver microsomes, for example, after treatment with AAPH[43]. Similarly, Pc protects red blood cells against lysis induced by peroxyl radicals[44].

In vivo oxidation often leads to inflammation, and antioxidant action is often associated with similar anti-inflammatory effects. This is also true for Pc. A typical model to test the effects of agents like Pc, involves injecting glucose oxidase into the paws of test mice. This enzyme reacts with endogenous glucose to produce local hydrogen peroxide that dissociates to form hydroxyl radicals. Together, these cause tissue damage and accompanying inflammatory changes[45]. Phycocyanin has been shown to significantly reduce mouse paw edema in a dose dependent fashion[41]. The scavenging of the hydroxyl radicals is presumed to account, at least in part, for the anti-inflammatory effects observed. Other inflammatory methods for causing similar paw edema, involving arachidonic acid or carageenan which both manifest different pathways of inflammation, were also shown to be inhibited by Pc[46,47].

Enough said. The fact that Pc shows antioxidant and anti-inflammatory effects, is a potential positive side effect of consuming AFA. But that is really only a side show that adds to the main drama that remains our focus in this book, namely Stem Cell Nutrition. That's the main thing and someone else has rightly admonished that one should 'always let the main thing be the main thing'.

However, this is by no means the whole story. Nature has its own agenda. Scientists and researchers are only invited to the party as guests. Some privileges are restricted even though the party goes on. There is much that happens naturally in biology (and more specifically, physiology) that we still do not understand. But the atoms, molecules and cells etc. go about their daily tasks of supporting life and promoting health even when we are unaware of the details of their behavior.

Thus Stem Cell Nutrition, being a natural dietary intervention, introduces packages of nutrients and other ingredients that have a wide array of physiological benefits that derive not from research and understanding on our part, but from their intrinsic properties and the synergy of nature's way.

We have not taken the time to describe here, for example, the effect of the polyunsaturated fatty acids (PUFA) in AFA on the lipid profile as seen in animal studies[48]. This positive hypocholesterolemic effect is suggestive of a possible benefit in this regard, with human consumption. Then there are the further benefits to be derived from chlorophyll, trace minerals and other ingredients.

There are probably benefits to be experienced before they are explained. But that remains as no excuse for either negligence or indifference to the call of science and research to investigate further, if only to gain better control for future health optimization and wellness promotion. That is a call still worth heeding.

12-Point
SUMMARY OF PART TWO

1. The food supply has become industrialized and advertising and modern lifestyles have shifted dietary choices away from wholesome natural food. Therefore, supplementation represents the wise alternative to guarantee an adequate supply of essential nutrients, on a daily basis and in a convenient form.

2. During the last century, as the understanding of the role of nutrition in human physiology has increased, there has been a growing list of dietary supplements that have proven to be effective in the pursuit of optimum health and wellness. That list includes vitamins, essential fatty acids, herbal products, fiber, antioxidants, digestive enzymes, nutrient delivery systems and more.

3. Algae provide some rich sources of essential nutrients and there has been a long tradition of anecdotal evidence of health benefits associated with the safe consumption of edible algae. Microalgae, especially Aphanizomenon flos aquae(AFA) , harvested in the wild from a prestine region in the Pacific Northwest of the US, has developed a reputation for health benefits, consistent with substantial research studies, both *in vitro* and *in vivo*. Similar statements can be made regarding fucoidan derived from macroalgae, especially *Undaria Pinnatifida*, harvested in the wild from prestine regions in Tasmania and Petagoria.

4. In pursuit of some mechanism(s) by which AFA could exert such a variety of benefits to consumers, researchers first found that consumption of AFA leads to rapid changes in immune

cell trafficking. There was no direct activation of lymphocytes. In this way, AFA increases immune surveillance – (lymphocytes and monocytes, but not polymorph nucleated cells).

5.   A water soluble extract of AFA was shown to directly activate NK cells *in vitro* and to modulate the chemokine receptor profile. In particular, the down regulation of CXCR4 may reduce homing of NK cells to the bone marrow environment. But at the same time, the NK cells probably become more sensitive to other chemotactic signals that increase homing to other tissues as part of general immune surveillance. Other studies show a potent immune-stimulatory effect of a high molecular weight polysaccharide fraction from AFA. These combined results could account for observed (immuno-modulating) benefits from AFA *in vivo*.

6.   The presence of Phycocyanin as one of the major pigment constituents, probably accounts for the observed anti-oxidant and anti inflammatory effects observed with AFA consumption in moderate amounts (as is typical for dietary supplementation).

7.   The common anecdotal reports of elevated mood, improved focus, attention and concentration with AFA consumption, have been attributed to the presence of phenylethylamine (PEA). This is a naturally occurring alkaloid that is known as an important neuromodulator or neurotransmitter. The short half life of pure ingested PEA casts doubts on these effects, but it could very well be that the natural whole food is exerting an influence in concert, surpassing the effect of isolated PEA.

8.   Speaking of 'an influence in concert', the effects of AFA surpass all expectations because the natural product contains a variety of bioactive ingredients that go about their mission without any limitation or restriction from human knowledge

and understanding. All the players perform perfectly.

9.   As the research on the possible mechanisms of AFA action were being investigated, and while reviewing the relevant literature, a new hypothesis emerged. Christian Drapeau and Dr. Gitte S. Jensen proposed that the body has a natural healing and renewal system, whereby adult stem cells are constantly being released from the bone marrow. They then traffick under the influence of chemokines to affected tissues in need, whereupon they migrate into those tissues, then they proliferate and differentiate to become cells of the particular tissue(s).

10.   Published research from many centers has provided increasing evidence to support the hypothesis. It is now becoming more generally accepted that the number of circulating stem cells is another appropriate marker for overall disease risk and a determinant of health outcomes.

11.   Drapeau and Jensen then proved that the consumption of an AFA extract, conveniently enriched for the important L-selectin ligand, was effective in enhancing the otherwise normal release of adult stem cells from the bone marrow by as much as 20-30 percent. Similar results were also found from the consumption of fucoidan derived from a specific concentration of *Undaria Pinnatifida*. This dietary intervention can therefore improve the maintenance, regeneration and repair of tissues, when and as required.

12.   This Stem Cell Nutrition that can support the normal release, circulation and migration of adult stem cells now represents the leading edge of nutrition and affords a new innovative strategy to promote optimal health and wellness.

Who would have imagined that an ingredient in a common micro-algae (cyanobacteria) like *aphanizomenon flos-aquae* (AFA) could have such a significant impact on the normal renewal system of the human body. That is a most unusual source of such physiological innovation. That's what we are about to discover in **Part Three** which follows on immediately.

But AFA is as unique as it is convenient and totally natural. After all, that's what nature typically does. As we have observed several times before, nature tends to provide solutions to meet nature's needs. This is just one more illustration of that consistent phenomenon.

So, in Chapter 7 we will explore the unique circumstances that create the idyllic situation for the conversion of 'pond scum' to 'pure nutritional gold'. Later we will describe the methods for harvesting and processing this 'gold', while maintaining standards of excellence that guarantee quality and safety. That's all essential to effective **Stem Cell Nutrition.**

Part III

Sources of Innovation

innovation: *formation and exploitation of new ideas; a process of renewal or change; a new value-added solution to market needs; creativity*

Preamble to Part Three

We live in an age that is driven by technology. Since the last World War, innovations in science and technology have transformed the way we live in unmistakable ways. Consider the industrialized food we eat to sustain our bodies, the practice of high-tech medicine to repair those same bodies, the instantaneous dissemination of information, the speed of travel and the inescapable presence of media and entertainment. All this and much more has changed modern lives and lifestyles in a way that would be inconceivable to our great grandparents.

The late great Steve Jobs was an American entrepreneur who became clearly a master innovator of his generation. As the Co-founder, Chairman and CEO of *Apple Inc.*, he spearheaded a revolution in the application of personal computers, among other things. He oversaw the development of the *iMac, iTunes, iPod, iPhone* and *iPad* and caused a broad transformation in the way we receive, utilize and retransmit all types of information. His innovations directed the way the world now chooses to live, to work and to play. His was an inescapable testimony to the power of innovation. He led and the world followed – a modern Pied Piper indeed.

The concept of innovation is probably readily understood by all, when Steve Jobs' career is the illustration at hand. But it is not as clear when one tries to define it unambiguously. It is not exactly the same as inventiveness or even creativity.

Inventiveness or creativity emphasizes the birth of a new idea, the origination of a new method, the design of a new gadget of some kind that does something else, something more, something better. It begins somewhere and goes from there. But that misses a key element. Innovation is best appreciated as the ability or the process of doing something different or unusual, something unanticipated. It is not just an improvement of some prior thing or some prior idea that makes it better – it is more the evolution of a new thing, a fundamental change in *modus operandus* (or *modus conceptus*, if you like) that leads to change or transformation, with a kind of inherent discontinuity.

This is innovation at its best. But let's take the concept just a step further before we return to Stem Cell Nutrition.

Innovation clearly has widespread effects. In society, it enhances every aspect of daily life – hopefully increasing comfort, indulging convenience and improving efficiency in every area. In business and commerce, innovation is the catalyst to growth, especially in the midst of technological change. Great entrepreneurs (like Steve Jobs was), are always looking for alternative ways, different methods, better applications, organizational changes, new strategies, creative initiatives, – in a word 'innovations' that generate the emerging technologies which inevitably, with time, grow to surpass whatever exists before. They drive the cutting edge of societal evolution.

But not so fast. Clearly, most technical innovation comes about by research and development (so-called R & D). Almost every significant business, often independent of their particular product or service, finds that to remain competitive, they must invest in research and development. They anticipate that innovations will come as an end-product of that R & D process. And that is generally true, with notable exceptions of serendipity, just plain 'luck' or 'good fortune'. The big 'breakthroughs'- in industry, engineering, medicine, even government – have by and large come about by deliberate research efforts. These efforts have not necessarily been targeted to specific results or applications. But in a process of inquiry and investigation, they have followed ideas where they led and let results dictate the future activities. That's the story of science and technology. That's how man walked on the moon, developed the internet or cured infectious disease.

But that's still not the whole picture. Many incremental but important innovations have come about, not from research labs, but from the daily life and lifestyle practice that stumbled upon new creative applications that were unanticipated but clearly significant. Stem Cell Nutrition is such an innovation.

No researcher set out a *priori* to find a way to utilize common natural products to enhance stem cell release. No one devised some equation or formula that predicted that there was anything edible on the face of the earth that would be selective for ligands or cell surface receptors in the human bone marrow. For a very long time, no one even considered that stem cells were so important – especially adult stem cells. Even in the face of active and specialized investigation of cell differentiation and proliferation, the concept of a natural renewal system based on the normal release of stem cells from bone marrow was not only obscure, it was (and still is to some professionals) ridiculous.

So, this innovation of Stem Cell Nutrition has truly come about, in some ways, backwards. Here was a fairly common blue green algae that had been consumed for centuries in different parts of the world. Here was a natural product that was reputed to have quite amazing health benefits when consumed, originally with no known physiological explanation. Ordinary people were consuming AFA and experiencing changes to their health (at least, that was their anecdotal experience). They knew nothing of stem cells -- nothing of bone marrow release, nothing of cell migration and homing to tissues, nothing of differentiation and proliferation. But in reality, they were experiencing Stem Cell Nutrition. They were experiencing innovation from nature. Here was innovation being reported, not by the originator, but by the end-user. The innovation was not in ideas but in experience. The source of that innovation was not an R & D laboratory, but the crucible of human experience. It was safe, it was effective and it was real.

That is the story of nature. **Intrinsic to nature is the supply of essentials for normal human life.** With the passage of time and experience, we have become informed of nature's secrets. Those are secrets to us, but nature is never ignorant of its own potential. Essential nutrients have always been exactly that, no more and no less. Long before we discovered the existence of vitamins, for example, humans have consumed citrus fruits and rosehips replete with vitamin C. We later learned that ascorbic acid does have a myriad of functions in the human cell. But every single vitamin C molecule that ever entered there 'knew' exactly what it had to do. By Intelligent Design, all the nutrient molecules have intrinsic characteristics ideally suited to fulfill their destiny. They do that whether we have knowledge of their activity or not. We never teach the nutrients themselves, we only educate the students of nutrition (and sometimes reluctant or even resistant professionals) who need to learn. The nutrients on the other hand, just go about their daily business, doing what they do best ... applying the finest principles of physiology and biochemistry to enhance health and well-being. That's incredible, but true.

So Stem Cell Nutrition arose, naturally and spontaneously, more by unintended default than by human craftiness. And it began with a most unlikely candidate for a major role in the nutrition drama. Such is *Aphanizomenon flos-aquae*, (AFA) sometimes described in not so flattering terms as "pond scum". How ironic and how disengaged from reality that is, when we consider its value as an ancient food. It must utter silent screams of verbal injustice every time the uninformed uses such derogatory language. Because this common, ordinary, unassuming and unattractive algae –this 'living flower of the water'- just happens to be a species of cyanobacteria that constitutes one of the most complete foods on the face of the earth. Just think of this: AFA contains a spectrum of more than 60 micronutrients including:

Table 1. Nutrients in Aphanizomenon flos aquae

Glyco-proteins	12 Vitamins
Simple carbohydrates	27 Essential minerals
Polysaccharides	11 Pigments
Omega-3 fatty acids	Phycoyanin
Lipids	Beta carotene
Phenylethylamine(PEA)	Biologically active enzymes

We have only recently begun to appreciate the nutritional value of each of these nutrients. They do wonders for the human body and as we learn more, we discover their intrinsic worth, even if we do not always know how they do what they do. **Nutrition remains a young science and if that's in infancy, then Stem Cell Nutrition is a true neonate.**

In the next Chapter, we will explore in some detail the *sources* of AFA in its natural habitat – a pristine environment of pure beauty. We will see how it came to be such an amazing food product and a remarkable innovation in Stem Cell Nutrition. We'll go on in Chapter 8 to describe the basic details of *harvesting and processing* the AFA that blooms in abundance each year. Then in Chapter 9, we will address the very important issues of *quality, food safety and toxicity.* There is so much to appreciate about such an unlikely source of innovation, the innovation we now correctly describe as **Stem Cell Nutrition.**

CHAPTER 7

From Pond Scum
to Pure Gold

Historically, the use of algae as a source of food** and as traditional treatment for a variety of physical ailments goes back thousands of years. In the Far East, evidence exists confirming the use of seaweed (macroalgae) for food as far back as 6000 BC. (To put that in context, recorded history involving the use of language began only about 4000 BC). There is also evidence that by about 900 AD, many species of algae were suitable not only as food, but also as a form of primitive medical treatment.

BASIC ALGOLOGY

The term 'algae' in common usage tends to be an all-inclusive designation for the similar organisms found growing freely on the surface of bodies of water, in water columns or sometimes even in terrestrial environments on snow or ice. However, in reality, there are thousands of different known species and they differ in a multitude of ways. The modern study of marine and fresh water algae – known as *Algology* (Latin) or *Phycology* (Greek) – has become highly sophisticated. The subject is vast but certainly worthy of mention before we delve into the important blue-green algae or cyanobacteria, *Aphanizomenon flos-aquae* (AFA). That is the focus of our attention here.

Although the singular term *alga* (Latin) is the more appropriate word for any particular seaweed, we will continue to use the common plural designation *algae*, even in reference to the various species individually. That's more for convenience than anything else. Further, the actual cyanobacteria which are referred to loosely as blue-green algae, are formally not algae at all. This latter term is now technically restricted to *eukaryotic* organisms which all have defined nuclei enclosed within membranes. The cyanobacteria in question, on the other hand, are *prokaryotic*, (that is, without defined nuclei) and are more correctly regarded as bacteria. That distinction in classification is really a moot point in the context of this book, one which is intended to be a tutorial open to all and not a thesis.

In general though, algae are a very large and diverse group of simple organisms that vary from invisible unicellular microscopic forms like *phytoplankton*, to multi-cellular forms that are many meters in length. They carry out photosynthesis by converting carbon dioxide and water, in the presence of light energy and minerals (as catalysts), into glucose and oxygen. As the algae grow and multiply, they incorporate a wide variety of nutrients other than glucose, which makes them a convenient source of nutrition not only for marine life, but also for human consumption.

But not all algae are safe to eat. Most of the edible algae is that which is commonly found as seaweed (marine algae). In contrast, most freshwater algae tend to be toxic. Those are general statements only, and again, major exceptions exist in either case. Here's a short list of the most common edible algae known and utilized in different parts of the world: [1]

Table 2.   Edible Algae

- Aphanizomenon flos-aquae
- Arame
- Badderlocks
- Bladderwrack
- Carola
- Carrageenan moss
- Channeled wrack
- Chlorella
- Cochayuyo
- Dulse
- Eucheuma
- Gelidiella
- Gracilaria
- Gutweed
- Hijiki or Hiziki
- Hypnea
- Irish moss
- Laver
- Limu Kala
- Kombu
- Mozuku
- Nori
- Oarweed
- Ogonori
- Sugar kelp
- Sea Grapes or green caviar
- Sargassum
- Sea lettuce
- Spiral wrack
- Spirulina
- Thongweed
- Wakame

To illustrate the value and use of edible seaweed in general, we'll just take a cursory look at three popular *macroalgae* (seaweed) and three important *microalgae* (including cyanobacteria) to help put 'algae as food' in proper context. We begin with the macroalgae, typically referred to as 'seaweed'.

EDIBLE SEAWEED

Seaweeds are utilized quite extensively as food in many coastal areas around the world. Particularly in the Far East, they have been a regular part of the common diets in China, Japan and Korea since prehistoric times. But they have also made their way into many traditional European kitchens (for example, in Iceland, Norway and the Atlantic coast of France), into Northwestern Ireland, Wales, Southwest England and Atlantic Canada. Nevertheless, it is fair to observe that whereas seaweeds have been highly valued by Oriental communities for thousands of years and remain so today, no such tastes or traditions have widely caught on in the West. The Greeks and Romans had little regard for seaweed as food, and the use of algae as a specific food item has been frowned on and is still avoided in most of Europe and North America. But there really has been little or no justification for this dietary prejudice. Discretion is usually the better part of valor, but this indiscretion has proven to be the greater part of nutritional folly.

Let's take a closer look. Three of the most widely known seaweeds used for food today are: *Porphyra, Laminaria* and *Undaria pinnatifida*. Together these three constitute the vast majority of all the edible algae being consumed anywhere today. We'll consider each of them in turn.

Porphyra

This is the most widely consumed edible seaweed in the world.

Most ethnic groups with access to *Porphyra*, use it in some form in the diet, making it perhaps the most domesticated of all the marine algae. It grows in cold shallow sea water and has been harvested as a vegetable in Southeast Asia for well over a thousand years. This red algae is comprised of about 70 different species. It is harvested and processed mainly to make dry thin sheets that are used primarily to wrap sushi and as a garnish or flavoring in noodle preparations and soups in Asian cuisine. In Japan, the most popular product by far is *nori*, the typical sushi wrap for rice and fish. They also make it into a toasted variety (*ajitsuke-nori*), flavoring it with soy sauce, spices, sugar and other condiments. In China, they call it *zicai* which is used not only as food but in traditional Chinese medicine as an aid in treatment of goiter, beriberi, edema, urinary infection and sore throat. In Korea, it is referred to as *gim* which is often used as a side dish after it is toasted with sesame oil, sprinkled with fine salt and cut into squares. Sometimes *gim* is made into very fine sheets and used in the original dry state without being roasted. Actually, porphyra products tend to easily absorb water from the air and degrade, so it is very important to use a desiccant to keep it dry during storage. In recent time, annual production in Japan alone is about 250 – 400,000 tons from some 230 square miles of coastal waters, with an economic value that exceeds US $1 billion. This is therefore not an insignificant part of their food industry[2].

The Chinese produce about one-third of that, using some fairly sophisticated methods. In one typical agricultural method, for example, Porphyra spores are sprinkled on oyster shells which are then placed into shallow tanks. The spores germinate to form tiny filaments on these shells. In turn, these early filaments produce their own spores which are then caught on strings dipped into the tank. These strings are then placed in shallow bays. After about two months the algae plants become fully grown on the strings from which they are then stripped and dried in the sun. Alternately, repeated seeding is done on the sea surface and the first harvest takes place after about 45 days, even though the plants themselves grow quite rapidly. These algae farmers typically use nets suspended from boats and then do mechanical harvesting with a variety of configurations. They collect several harvests from each seeding, at about ten day intervals. The raw product is then processed by fairly automated machines that more or less duplicate the traditional manual techniques. That improves efficiency and consistency.

Speaking of consistency, *Porphyra* has been imported to North America from Japan and China for about fifty years, but the products available in health food stores and Asian-American grocery stores vary widely. The price alone reflects that. A sheet of *nori* can sell anywhere from about a nickel to a dollar, and customers tend to get what they pay for.

Nonetheless, *Nori* is quite nutritious. It is about one third protein and one third dietary fiber. It contains high proportions of iodine, carotene, vitamins A, B and C, as well as significant amounts of calcium, iron and other trace nutrients.

Laminaria

This seaweed is commonly referred to as 'kelp' and represents some 31 different species of brown algae. It grows quite large and is characterized by its long, leathery laminae (hence, its name). Again, it is widely eaten in Southeast Asia. In Japan, it is known as *Kombu, in* China as *kunbu* or *kaida;* and in Korea as *dashima or dasima.*

This edible brown algae grows to depths of almost 100 feet in the Southeast Asian waters as well as in the northern Atlantic Ocean and the northern Pacific Ocean. It is a very popular seaweed in Japan where it is used as an 'all-purpose' product but especially as an ingredient in bean-curd soup. Served in a variety of ways, it can be eaten fresh on sashimi, made into soup stock like *dashi* by simply adding it to cold water and bringing to a near boil, or diced and simmered in soy sauce and *mirin* to make *tsukudari*. It may also be pickled with sweet and sour flavoring, then cut into strips to make an accompaniment to green tea as a delicious snack. By itself it can be added to water as a dried or powdered *kombu* and brewed to make seaweed tea. South Koreans also process this kelp into a sweet meat known as *laminaria jelly*, in addition of course, to the popular *dashima* flavored soups.

From a nutritional perspective, this Asian kelp is a good source of the amino acid, glutamic acid or glutamate. Physiologically, glutamic acid is one of the three amino acids that constitute glutathione the principal intracellular antioxidant. Kelp is also well known to contain iodine, which is essential for normal growth and development. It is also a source of dietary fiber.

Again, this brown kelp has found a place in traditional Chinese medicine associated with treatments of goiter, tumor, edema, and surprisingly, testicular pain and swelling. Interestingly, *Laminaria* has been at times used to help dilate the cervix when necessary. Presumably the kelp would absorb moisture and then expand, thereby subsequently expanding the cervix. Clearly, this would not be an ideal practice in an age of modern medicine, particularly here in the West.

Traditionally, wild *Lamanaria* seaweed has been collected manually and then prepared in a variety of ways for human consumption. However, in the last century, methods of deliberate cultivation have been exploited so that today the product is made inexpensively and is therefore readily available. The Japanese produce over 150,000 tons per year and the Chinese have been reported to produce even more. In North America, it is also available as a dry edible food in health and Asian-American grocery stores.

Undaria pinnatifida

This is another brown seaweed or kelp that is smaller in size than *Laminaria*. It is an annual species that grows typically around two to four feet in length but can mature up to about 10 feet. It is native to the Sea of Japan, particularly in coastal areas west of Hokkaido, the coasts of Korea and in some parts of China. It was accidentally introduced to the Mediterranean about 1970 and has since accumulated in the waters off the coasts of France, Britain, the Netherlands, Spain and Italy. It has also proliferated in parts of South America and as far as Australia and New Zealand.

Undaria pinnatifida inhabits the inter-tidal zone down to the sub tidal zone, to a depth of some 40-60 feet in clear waters. It is found mainly in sheltered reef areas that are subject to oceanic influence, but rarely in highly exposed areas. It has been collected from these natural habitats for centuries and today is aggressively harvested mainly on ropes, between February and June. It is dragged ashore by long hooks, then washed in fresh water and dried. Production is in the hundreds of thousands of tons in Japan and Korea, but is much lower in China where *Laminaria* harvesting is dominant. *Undaria* is a highly invasive and hardy species, which grows so rapidly that it tends to overwhelm and exclude other native algal species. Sometimes seen as an opportunistic weed, it can at times be a nuisance contaminant in other marine farms. It is also known to spread by fouling ship hulls. On the California coastline it has become an economic and ecological threat to basically every industry there, so much so that marine biologists and other scientists are aggressively working to contain, if not totally remove it, to protect the treasured coastline.

As a food, *Undaria* is consumed, again, mainly in Asian cuisine. In Japan, it is commonly eaten as a sea vegetable called *Wakame*, in Korea it is known as *Miyeok*, whereas in China it is the less common *gundai cai.*

Wakame is generally distributed either dried or salted and finds its main culinary applications in soups (especially the ever popular Japanese miso soup) and in salads (mainly the delicate tofu salad). It is also served as a side dish with tofu, mixed with other salad vegetables like cucumber or by itself, simply sprinkled with sesame. These side dishes may be dressed with soy sauce and/or vinegar/rice vinegar.

Wakame is rich in several nutrients including iodine, essential fatty acids, a carotenoid called fucoxanthin, as well as several trace and ultra-trace elements. Some research reports have associated potential anti-viral[3] and antioxidant[4] activity with sulphated polyanions and polysaccharide fractions that are derivatives of Wakame. Studies in mice have shown that fucoxanthin induces the expression of a fat-burning protein (called UCPI) that accumulates in fatty tissue around internal organs[5]. As such this has prompted the promotion of wakame as an aid to human weight loss programs, but as of yet no clear evidence of effectiveness in humans has been presented.

In traditional Chinese medicine, *Undaria* has been associated with treatments for blood purification, intestinal strength, skin, hair, reproductive organs and menstrual regularity. Korea has an interesting tradition. The soup made from *miyeok* is frequently consumed by women during pregnancy and after giving birth. And then, the same preparation is traditionally eaten on birthdays as a reminder of the first food that the mother had eaten and passed on to her newborn through her breast milk. This ritual is presumed to bring good fortune throughout the following year.

Of particular note here, it is important to point out that of all the macroalgae, *Undaria* is the only one known to significantly support the release of stem cells from the bone marrow. This of course relates to its fucoidan content as we saw back in the previous chapter.

In North America, *Undaria* is consumed almost exclusively as wakame, which is frequently served in Japanese restaurants and sushi bars. The dried product is imported and can be readily found, again in health food and Asian American grocery stores.

In summary, edible seaweeds (macroalgae) have established a prominent place particularly in Asian cuisine, especially in Japan and to a somewhat lesser extent, in China and Korea. Their safe consumption has been justified over thousands of years and they are more popular today, not only in Asia but around the world. Perhaps there are influences of culture and taste that limit more widespread acceptance of this seaweed (algae) as food. Of interest only here, there may also be a physiological factor. Researchers have found bacterial enzymes in the digestive tract of Japanese that they failed to find in the North American population. It has been theorized that this phenomenon is probably a result of secondary transfer from the marine bacteria over time rather than an intrinsic genetic difference[6].

We have also noted that edible seaweed provides good sources of several important nutrients, including iodine, calcium, protein, vitamins, essential fatty acids and soluble fiber. These algae have also had a role in traditional Chinese medicine for centuries but there has been little pharmaceutical exploitation of these associations. This is partly understandable. The drug companies are attracted to smaller well characterized molecules that can be more readily synthesized, isolated and refined, or even modified neatly and reproducibly. Macromolecules tend be more challenging and intractable.

Perhaps it will be left to the microalgae to make dramatic breakthrough in the health benefits and even clinical applications in the

West. Good basic science and effective clinical trials are irresistible even in an age of modern medicine. So let's see where we are with the microalgae and what innovations are taking place.

MICROALGAE AS FOOD

It is really no big surprise that some macroalgae became part of the normal diet, even if that occurred mainly in Southeast Asia. Obviously the seaweed was there, and visibly so. The plants were large enough to attract attention and sooner or later it was probably observed that some marine (animals) organisms were living on a seaweed diet. It was right there for the taking and easy for humans to collect. There was the temptation at least to try it, to see if one would like it. If it was not eaten immediately, it could be dried and preserved for later, so that way it could be easily stored and transported. If 'the taste is in the pudding', the seaweed turned out to be both palatable and nutritious, so it was likely to become a shared experience. Soon the nutritional value would be recognized, especially as a source of iodine to avoid noticeable incidence of goiter, by experience. This seaweed then became a food and later made its way into traditional Chinese medicine. It turned out to be safe, delicious and effective, at least in that part of the world. If history and geography determined its origins as food, then as travel and commerce expanded, those same factors would introduce the edible seaweeds to the cuisines and dining tables around the world. And that they have.

Not so with the microalgae. Their story would be entirely different. These smaller, generally unicellular organisms, tend to appear as phytoplankton in marine systems, dispersed as a cloudy suspension in fresh water (ponds, lakes, rivers) or else accumulated on the surface as unattractive 'scum' that hardly invites the appetite to engage. But sometimes nature dictates that necessity be the mother of discovery and invention, even if or when experimentation is only justified by trial and error. Indeed, population pressure and famine have always been and still are forces which cause normal people to exploit most living things as possible sources of food as well as narcotic[7]. That may rationalize the original attempts to eat this 'pond scum', at least in the few areas where it was somewhat driven by necessity and not sensual appeal.

Perhaps it began in the Americas. In a glimpse at Aztec food technology, Farrer described how the Spanish used microalgae as staple food back in the sixteenth century[8]. When the Conquistadores reached Tenochtitlan, the capital of the old Aztec Empire and the site of what has become present day Mexico City, they found a large population of over 250,000, exceeding even the large European towns that they had known and left behind. The South American city was actually situated on an island in Lake Texcoco which had non-potable brackish water. The inhabitants got their fresh water from springs on the island and also via an aqueduct from the mainland. They got fish from the lake and on land they cultivated low-yielding maize, but they still had no domesticated animals suitable for food. These settlers resorted to collecting the 'scum' off the lake, drying it in the sun and making it into hard cakes that they not only consumed but also sold to others. This food they called *Tecuitlatl*, which reportedly tasted somewhat like cheese. This cake was made even more delicious by adding a pungent sauce that they called *Chilmolli*. So, this lake scum that served the population at that time is generally agreed to be blue-green algae, which we now know to be nothing else but cyanobacteria otherwise referred to as spirulina!

Across the Atlantic Ocean, around Lake Chad in Central Africa, French Colonial Troops found almost 100 years ago, a popular food-stuff called 'die' which turned out to be a mass of spiral filaments of blue green algae, since then identified as indeed, spirulina[7]. The algae grow in shallow ponds located in Wadis. After being collected in big baskets, the water was decanted and the remaining algae sundried as large 1 cm thick cakes. It was a rather exotic food used for making soup and formed a jelly-like mass in water. Others have identified a similar food item north-east of Lake Chad, called '*Dihe*' or '*Douhe*' which again turns out to be 'spirulina cakes'. Dihe smells like dried fish and has a slightly salty taste. The cakes are usually broken into pieces and soaked in water, then mixed with pimento, a pinch of salt and made into a nourishing soup, with or without added pieces of meat. Alternatively, dihe makes a very thick gravy used for seasoning millet made into balls. Tribesmen in Central Africa have valued these edible products as a weaning food for infant children (consistent with what we now know of them as a good source of vitamins).

The Russians and Chinese have used edible algae going back hundreds of years. *Nostoc edule*, for example, does not occur free-floating on the surface as 'scum', but can be found in large masses at the bottom of rivers, lakes and swamps[7]. It is very popular in the northern parts of Russia as well as in Mongolia and China. It is a highly esteemed ingredient in soups. The Chinese make it as a special treat on feast days and other celebratory occasions. In contrast, *Nostoc commune* is a different alga that is found free-lying on the soil as convoluted small pellets all over Europe and the Asiatic far North. They are eaten locally after boiling with meat and other additives. In Ecuador, this algae species called '*Yuyucho*', is boiled and eaten with garden vegetables just as others in Fiji and Okinawa have done– which brings us again to the Japanese.

In the very mountainous regions of southern Japan, villagers have used nets to gather a different type of blue-green algae called 'suizenji-nori (technically, *Phylloderma sacrum*). They do this all year round but the bulk of the harvesting is done mainly in the summer months. After removing other adhering algae, they cut the mass of colonies into small pieces which they spread on rocks and dry in the sun[9]. This forms sheets of edible algae, a product that can still be bought in Japan today, but since it is relatively rare and somewhat exotic, it is regarded nowadays as an expensive delicacy.

In reality, microalgae represent a novel ingredient in Western nutrition. For centuries they have been known and utilized as food in other parts of the world, mostly out of desperation in local isolated communities, but with little widespread acceptance. Now that some of these have been found to possess rich nutritional ingredients, they have become more acceptable and more readily available, thanks to commercial large-scale production and harvesting.

Most commercial producers of microalgae are located in the Asia-Pacific Rim. More than 100 commercial producers have an annual production capacity in the range of 300-500,000 tons. They cultivate a variety of microalgae including *Chlorella, Spirulina, Dunaliella, Tetraselmis, Skeletonema, Isochrysis, Nannochloropsis, Nitzschia, Crypthecodinium and Chaetoceros*[10].

Of the many thousands of known microalgae species (including more generally, the cyanobacteria), only a few have found any significant place in the contemporary normal diet. More precisely, they are used as dietary supplements for their presumed nutritional and/or health benefits. Three in particular attract our attention here. They are *Spirulina, Chlorella* and of course the star of this show-*Aphanizomenon flos-Aquae* (AFA). We'll comment on each of these in turn.

Spirulina

To be technically correct, spirulina is not a true microalga but is actually a cyanobacteria, made up primarily of two species: *Arthrospira platersis* and *Arthorspira maxima*. But what does it matter? The historical and popular present day association with other microalgae justifies its inclusion here. As we saw earlier, that was probably the stuff traditionally harvested from small lakes and ponds in the vicinity of Lake Chad in Central Africa.

It was also the same 'scum' that was used by the Meso-Americans, after being harvested from Lake Texcoco by the Aztecs, at least until the 16th century. It would appear that sometime after that, the surrounding feeder lakes were drained for agricultural and urban development. Much later, a mere 40 years ago, a large scale spirulina production plant was eventually introduced back in that area.

In the past few decades commercial operations have sprung up in places like the US, China, India, Taiwan, Pakistan, Thailand, Greece, Chile and Myanmar. Today, spirulina is hardly harvested from the wild. It is typically cultivated in open channel raceway ponds, with paddle wheels that agitate the water. That water environment is strategically controlled for temperature, pH, carbon dioxide and minerals to optimize yields. It is harvested and processed into dry tablets, flakes or powder, for use most commonly as a dietary supplement. It has also found market acceptance as a feed supplement in the aquaculture industry as well as in the aquarium and poultry industries. Today, estimates of annual production of spirulina exceed 2 million kilograms (4.4. million pounds) by dry weight.

The Spirulina itself consists of free-floating filamentous cyanobacteria (recognized as blue-green algae) characterized by cylindrical, multi-cellular trichomas in an open left hand helix. The *A. platensis* variety is found wild in Africa, Asia and South America, while the alternate *A. maxima* is apparently confined to Central America.

Spirulina has turned out to be a rather nutrient dense food. The dry product contains about 60% protein which is fairly complete in all the essential amino acids, except for insufficient methionine. Compared to other plant protein sources like legumes, it is outstanding. It has good lipid content (7% by weight) and is rich in several essential fatty acids. Spirulina also contains most B vitamins, as well as vitamins A, C, D and E. It is also a source of essential minerals and a number of beneficial pigments like beta-carotene, phyco-cyanin, chlorophyll and others.

Spirulina has attracted some research interest and in recent times, it has been the subject of preliminary human studies, in addition to *in vitro* and animal studies. *In vitro*, the potential activity against HIV[11] and its possible role as an iron-chelating agent[12] or radio-protective agent[13] have been examined. In animal studies, different researchers have investigated spirulina for possible influences in pre-vention of chemotherapy- induced heart damage,[14] stroke recov-ery,[15] age-related decline in memory,[16] diabetes mellitus,[17] ALS[18] and even rodent models of hay fever[19]. In humans, relative-ly small studies have looked at spirulina for malnourished chil-dren,[20] hay fever and allergic rhinitis,[21] hypertension[22] and for possibly improving exercise tolerance[23]. These studies should be considered preliminary and any therapeutic claims would be prema-ture and probably unjustified. The value of spirulina would be best appreciated today in its nutritional context. It is a source of food, or at least a food supplement and any other health benefit to be derived should be welcomed only as an unintended blessing, one in disguise and not by design. This would be totally consistent with the position taken by the US National Institutes of Health.

The US Food and Drug Administration (FDA) has designated spir-ulina to be 'generally recognized as safe' (GRAS) and rightly so. No significant adverse affects have been noted from spirulina consump-tion even after dozens of human clinical studies - including specific toxicology studies with relatively high doses[24]. The only caution-ary note would apply to patients taking anticoagulants because of the vitamin K content of spirulina, and those with a rare genetic disorder called PKU (phenylketonuria) since spirulina (like other high protein foods) contains an essential amino acid, phenylalanine, which they ought to avoid[25].

Before we leave the subject of spirulina, it is of interest to note that, thirty years ago, the space agencies in both the US and Europe considered spirulina as one of the primary foods to be cultivated during proposed long-term space missions. That proposal never took flight, but on a more down to earth level, a number of UN member states cooperated in an Intergovernmental Institution for the use of Micro-algae Spirulina Against Malnutrition (IIMSAM). This was an organized attempt to exploit the potential of spirulina in the 'sustainable development' agenda.

That latter initiative leads us directly to the second edible micro-algae that has quite a fascinating story.

Chlorella

The story of chlorella has two important and interesting lines. The first pertains to its pure nutritive value. Just consider that this microalgae has a composition of about 45% protein, 20% fat, 20% carbohydrate, 5% fiber and 10% minerals and vitamins, in addition to essential fatty acids. What a whole food that is.

In the middle of the last century, some concerned experts began to warn of an impending world-hunger crisis as the global population was growing uncontrollably and there was no apparent solution to the overwhelming problem of feeding the coming generations. Therefore, welcome to chlorella. Here was a new and promising primary food, suited for the teeming tropical environment. The prospect of producing astronomical amounts of chlorella as high quality food at relatively low cost captured the attention of powerful experts and stakeholders[26]. This micro-alga is very efficient at photosynthesis, it is inexpensive, easy to cultivate and harvest, and it requires little of the diminishing arable land which is also seen as another worldwide problem. It can be grown in warm, sunny, shallow conditions on water, in the tropics especially where it would probably be needed most.

Powerful established institutions got involved in chlorella research. Just look at this list: Stanford University, the US National Institutes of Health, Carnegie Institute, University of California at Berkeley, the Rockefeller Foundation and the Atlantic Energy Commission. That's not even the complete list of research participants in the push for a "chlorella solution" to world hunger at the time. In 1946 the UN Food and Agricultural Organization produced a report that concluded the world needed to produce one third more food between 1940 and 1960 just to keep up with the ballooning population. To reduce health consequences of malnutrition, food production would have to nearly double in that period.

Pilot research farms growing chlorella were initially quite promising and even the science media began to report with surprising exaggeration, that future populations of the world would be 'kept from starvation' by the production of new and improved algae. In other words, this green 'pond scum' could be cleaned up and sanitized to solve what they saw as a looming world hunger problem. Even more ambitious and elaborate was the idea that the common 'pond scum' would soon become the world's most import agricultural crop.

Then reality set in. Two things happened. What seemed so promising in a small laboratory proved disastrous when considered on a larger scale in the real world. Massive production facilities would need the use of artificial light and/or shade to maximize the efficiency of photosynthesis. Furthermore, the chlorella would require carbonated water for growth. Harvesting would be sophisticated and costly. Then, the material itself which has such tough cell walls that encapsulated nutrients would therefore need to be first pulverized before consumption. These and other challenges rained on the 'chlorella for commercial use' parade. It never really got on center stage. It could not even match spirulina, much less soybeans or whole grains. Costs alone killed the mega-idea.

The second big development was in the advances made in general agriculture that afforded better standard crop efficiency and yields. The massive crisis that had been predicted was averted (though not entirely) by the aggregate gains in agricultural science and economics. Today chlorella is at most a very minor, if not insignificant, player on the world agricultural stage. There went the rise and fall of a potential super food[26]. But who knows what is possible in the future?

The other interesting thing that has earned chlorella a place in history pertains to basic science. The Nobel Prize for Chemistry was awarded in 1961 to Melvin Calvin of the University of California, Berkeley. This was in recognition of his ground breaking work to unravel the process of photosynthesis. With chlorella as his 'subject' he used the newly discovered radioactive carbon isotope to trace the path of carbon assimilation in plants. He and his colleagues showed that sunlight acts on the chlorophyll pigment in a plant to fuel the manufacturing of organic compounds. Before this original carbon cycle was demonstrated, it was believed that the effect of sunlight was to act on the carbon dioxide directly.

The regal role of chlorella in plant photosynthesis goes back even further. Back in 1931, a German biochemist and cell physiologist Otto Heinrich Warburg, was awarded the Nobel Prize in Physiology or Medicine for his work on cell respiration. Not surprisingly perhaps. He too had used chlorella extensively in his research. So ironically, the chlorella microalgae gained recognition for its contribution to fundamental science, but it came up short on the path to glory when it was heralded as a superfood and 'panacea for world hunger', as it failed to deliver.

Nevertheless, chlorella is a true genus of single-cell green algae. Its name reflects its appearance (Greek: *chloros-* green and Latin: *ella -* small). It does indeed appear as a green microalgae, the importance of which ought not to be judged by size, for it packs a pretty punch. It has been used essentially as a food supplement because of its nutritional profile. Again, some small preliminary clinical studies in humans have suggested a possible role for chlorella as a detoxifier in the digestive tract, especially for heavy metals and some carcinogens[27,28]. It also appears to have some ability to reduce hypertension, lower serum cholesterol levels, accelerate wound healing and enhance immune functions[29]. Again, these limited trials should be regarded as preliminary and the value of chlorella would be better emphasized for its nutritional value rather than as a medicine.

There is nothing really fundamental here with the use of either spirulina or chlorella. There is no new innovation to expand the scope or understanding of human biology in any significant way. One could hardly make a case for any unusual empowerment of human cells, organs or tissues that make possible dramatic influences on human health. Still, it is fair to underscore the value of good nutrients that feed cells with important raw materials which help to optimize normal cellular activity and therefore promote good health and wellness. That's more than justifiable in its own right.

However, when we turn to our third microalgae exhibit, *Aphanizomenon flos aquae* (AFA) – the superstar of our show – we find something else. We do find a fundamental physiological system in the body that responds to its use as a dietary supplement. Recall our fundamental thesis: **Everybody has stem cells. Everybody uses stem cells. Everybody uses stem cells every day. Stem cells work ... and they work every time.** Therefore, since Stem Cell Nutrition enhances the normal release of stem cells from the bone marrow in a most convenient way, when we address this phenomenon we are dealing with a really different matter altogether.

So, let's go there.

Aphanizomenon flos-aquae (AFA)

AFA is really the newcomer on the algae block. It is the latest cyanobacterium (blue green algae) to be used as a food supplement, following the proven experience with spirulina and chlorella. It only came on to the commercial stage in the 1980's when it began to be harvested from the Pacific Northwest in the US. In less than two decades, the market for AFA exceeded US $100 million, with an annual production exceeding 1 million kilograms (2.2. million pounds) by dry weight[30].

The rise in AFA production and consumption is somewhat of a 'chicken-and-egg' story. The algae have been blooming on an historic lake for generations but until some brave resident or visitor was inclined to test the palatability of this 'pond scum', nothing happened. Now consider this scenario. Perhaps it took simple curiosity, suspicious error or sheer desperation to initiate the earliest ingestion of this prevalent algae when it was in full bloom on the lake surface. Perhaps also, some keen observer noted that waterfowl and predatory birds in the area were having a feast and coming back for more. Perhaps yet again, someone made an association with other blue green algae like spirulina and thought this was worth a try. Then the combination of satisfaction, safety and derived benefit would lead to repeated experimentation, then to cultural exchange and therefore spreading the word. This would then lead to further consumption, to acceptance and widespread use; to perceived benefit, to increased demand, to increased harvesting and increased availability, then to further demand. And the rest would be history.

The foregoing would be an example of consumption resulting in satisfaction, then satisfaction increasing demand, which leads to more harvesting and consumption. That becomes a spiral creating a market opportunity, which would be driven by further consumer demand. In this scenario, we would learn more about the natural product only as more consumers experience it. Therefore, it would be a case of consumer experience driving knowledge and understanding.

Now imagine an alternate scenario. Some entrepreneur becomes aware of this algae 'story'. Knowing about the reputation of other blue green algae like spirulina and/or chlorella, they perceive an opportunity. Commercial harvesting begins and a market for the product is pursued on the strength of spirulina's reputation, for example. As the market grows, other commercial harvesters get in on the action and competition stimulates further growth in terms of supply and demand. Now AFA is being consumed in significant quantities and anecdotes of health benefits begin to surface. These spread by word of mouth, increasing further demand.

Then at the turn of the century, researchers begin to look at AFA and its possible physiological effects. They discover the increased NK-cell activity, enhancing immune effects and relate that to the polysaccharides in AFA[31]. They discover the presence of phycocyanin and attribute the reported anti-inflammatory properties of AFA to that ingredient[32]. They further discover the presence of phenylethylamine (PEA) which could account for the testimonials of enhancements in mood, concentration and mental clarity[33]. But most of all, they surreptitiously find that an L-selectin ligand in AFA causes enhancement of stem cell release from the bone marrow[34]. That last effect is now credited with further supporting the body's natural renewal system with broad generalized consequences. That opens the flood gates as the innovation that is called Stem Cell Nutrition takes hold.

Now, in this latter scenario, knowledge can drive consumer experience and not vice versa, as in the first scenario above. Now the science of AFA can guide its use and application. Now the consumer can benefit by design and not by default. Now the message can be converted from 'try it, you might like it' to 'it works, so you should use it'. After all, remember that indeed **everybody has stem cells; everybody uses stem cells; everybody uses stem cells every day; stem cells work ... and they work every time.** That's the reality.

We have gone from 'pond scum' to 'pure gold'. This fresh water plant may have been considered previously as nothing more than a 'sore sight for the eyes'. It was regarded as an 'ecological nuisance' in an otherwise pristine environment. To local businesses, it was an economic spoiler deterring potential boaters and swimmers from enjoying the otherwise beautiful lake setting, while also distracting tourists and visitors. But now, that same undesirable AFA is known to be a precious commodity in the wild, just waiting for effective and environmentally sensitive commercial harvesting to be further expanded. Such an expansion would launch it on a broader journey that would hopefully terminate in its critical role of improving stem cell release from the bone marrow - an action that enhances the natural renewal process in living human bodies.

For that process to take place, it must be safely and efficiently brought to the consumer in whose hands it ultimately belongs. To that end, commercial harvesting is the subject of the next chapter.

CHAPTER 8

Harvesting
The Gold

phanizomenon flos-aquae (AFA) – this gold in disguise –
is not cultured in any controlled environment (in contrast to
Spirulina, for example). Rather, it is harvested in the wild
state from its normal pristine lake environment. There it grows in
natural abundance as part of an amazing ecosystem that has a most
interesting history and geography. Before describing the harvesting
procedures, we should explore these remarkable origins.

I am still awe-struck at the panorama I beheld when a good friend
took me on an excursion to this lake in the fall of 2012. It is a trip I
will remember for a very long time. The views were so incredibly
breathtaking and spectacular; I could have sat there forever in peaceful contemplation. That is an experience that I believe anyone else
would treasure.

A HABITAT OF BEAUTY

The visitors and tourists who come to the area of this lake each year
must often be heard to express their sense of awe and wonder as they
observe the beautiful natural topography in and around the Cascade
Mountain Range. Their experience does reach a climax at a higher
elevation, when they discover the large peaceful Crater Lake, resting
quietly in America's 5th National Park, established in 1902.

The vast deep blue lake sits serenely beneath multicolored lava walls that rise abruptly from the still water, as a silent testimony to a volcano's violent past. That was a very long time ago (perhaps about 7000 years) when geologists believe that Mt. Mazama erupted and sent flows of lava, pumice and ash all over the surrounding range. As a spectacular manifestation of forces which continue to shape the earth, Crater Lake furnishes compelling evidence of how volcanic activity built a mountain and then destroyed it through cataclysmic eruption. Much of what remained, collapsed to form a caldera that later filled (over time) from all the water run-off. Today Crater Lake is the deepest among all lakes in the United States and ranked 7th in the world, with a maximum depth of 1,943 ft. The awe-inspiring turquoise blue color reflects the clarity that allows visitors (especially amateur photographers looking for that perfect landscape opportunity) to see reflections in the water produced by the caldera walls. These reflections are visible at depths some 40 to 60 ft down. That happens routinely on summer days and on exceptional days even more amazing views to twice that depth have been enjoyed by some more fortunate tourists. A 33-mile scenic route called Rim Drive encircles the lake, allowing some 500,000 visitors each year to enjoy the immense beauty of this natural wonder.

Crater Lake may be the *pièce de résistance* of the region but the nutritional 'gold' is to be found in the much larger lake 50 miles to the south and just east of the Cascade Range. There we find Upper Klamath Lake, with a surface area of 61,543 acres, the largest fresh water lake in Oregon and one of the largest in the entire United States. It is a natural beauty in its own right, even though the overwhelming attraction of Crater Lake might often eclipse that observation.

The Cascade mountains create a rain shadow over much of the area, and precipitation varies between 15 – 50 inches each year, depending on the elevation. Therefore, the types of vegetation are quite diverse. In the more mountainous regions, there are forests of Douglas fir, ponderosa pine, lodge pole pine and true firs. However, on the open flatlands, there are mainly large pumice deposits where grasses and shrubs predominate. Throughout the wide drainage basin, there are large marshes. In particular, the Sycan Marsh and the Klamath Marsh cover relatively small basins which were former Pleistocene Lakes. They occupy as much as 995 acres and 8121 acres, respectively. These areas immediately surrounding Upper Klamath and Agency Lakes are almost exclusively marsh lands which typically support a sedge-reed community. Some of this marsh land has been reclaimed for agricultural use, progressively so since World War I. At the north edge of the lake sits the Upper Klamath National Wildlife Refuge. The entire area is a sanctuary for hundreds of species of resident and migrating wildlife.

There are several tributaries that feed into the lake. Some 17 visible rivers deposit an average of 50,000 tons of mineral-rich silt from the volcanic basin each year. Then there are many miles of underground rivers and streams that transport minerals from Crater Lake down to Upper Klamath Lake. The main tributary is the Williamson River that originates from a large spring and flows through pasture land before entering the Klamath marsh. It is joined by the smaller Sprague River, just before it enters the north end of the lake. At this point, it is a dark brown current of water, with high concentrations of dissolved aquatic humus (organic matter) and of course a wealth of minerals derived from all the volcanic deposits all over the area. That accounts for about half the tributary inflow.

The second largest tributary is the Wood River that drains into Agency Lake and subsequently into Upper Klamath Lake, again on the north shore. Other tributaries, which mostly drain agricultural areas, also enter the lake.

At the opposite end of the lake, to the south, water leaves the lake via the Link River that later becomes the Klamath River, which then goes all the way from Oregon through Northern California to empty into the Pacific Ocean.

As a water resource, Upper Klamath Lake serves south central Oregon in numerous ways:

- Water from the lake provides *supplemental irrigation* for reclaimed agricultural land.

- At the outflow end of the lake the water has been used to enhance *power generation* at the Pacific Power facilities on the Link River and further downstream at the John C. Boyle facility on the Klamath River

- During Spring and Fall migrations on the Pacific flyway, *waterfowl* use the marshy lands as an important stop over, the largest in the flyway.

- Fishing and boating on the lake are popular *recreational activities*.

- There are a number of resorts, campgrounds, picnic areas and boat launching sites strategically located around the lake, so this area is quite busy with *tourists*, especially during the summer.

Unlike Crater Lake, Upper Klamath Lake is relatively shallow. Most of it is less than 20 ft deep (the mean is 8ft) with a range extending to a maximum of about 60 ft. The deeper water seems more confined around the western shore.

The chemistry of the lake is also quite interesting, with the concentration of major aquatic ions and its conductivity slightly above average. The Williamson River brings a high concentration of phosphorus into the lake, derived from the natural springs and from surface run off. Therefore its concentration is quite high but obviously that varies with the season. The rather thick sediment at the bottom of the lake is not only rich in phosphorus but also in other important nutrients that help support the different life forms in the lake. There is also the unusual seasonal influx of dissolved organic matter from the marsh via the Williamson River.

Speaking of life forms, century-old records indicate that Upper Klamath Lake has always been very productive, supporting not only a huge *biomass* of algae, but also fish, waterfowl and birds. It has been a natural ecosystem quite diverse in its scope and somewhat ahead of its time. The earliest reports of collecting ice from the lake, going back to 1906, describe the ice as being green with algae. Lake suckers were so common that even novice fisherman could use pitchforks to harvest them. Ospreys were reported in densities up to 10 nests per square mile. Today there is still abundant activity and the Klamath Basin remains home to the largest congregation of bald eagles in the lower 48 states. These are all evidences of sustained life in the lake and surrounding area.

It is that same biomass on Upper Klamath Lake that got us to this point, for therein lies the star of our show, *Aphanizomenon flos-aquae* (AFA) - perhaps the most unlikely candidate to become the cornerstone of Stem Cell Nutrition today. But that it did. What natural innovation.

ALGAE ON THE LAKE

If one were to look for a reason why, despite all the natural beauty surrounding Upper Klamath Lake, there has never been much development on its shoreline, the key suspect would probably be that same biomass that blooms every summer. It appears as a natural but unwelcome 'contaminant' of the otherwise pristine environment. To that accusation, it would have to plead 'guilty as charged'. But before sentencing, it would redeem itself by virtue of what it provides ... a rich blessing in disguise. It now pleads for mercy and acceptance as a source of rare, natural L-selectin ligand that can enhance stem cell release from the bone marrow. The jury of proactive and well informed consumers must remember how this in turn favors the natural renewal system of the human body – a key determinant of optimum health and wellness in the 21st century. The court of public wellbeing repeatedly acknowledges that healthful claim and therefore responds with an honorable discharge: The microalgae may remain, proud and free. Case dismissed. Court adjourned.

Those blooms on the lake are completely natural and spontaneous. They are maintained from year to year by the rich nutrients springing up from the deposits at the bottom of the lake as well as the additional input originating in the surrounding marshes and delivered to the lake continuously by the Williamson River and all the other tributaries and springs. This has led to increased eutrophication ever since the lake's discovery by non-Native Americans, despite a number of significant changes. Eutrophication refers to the process by which bodies of water receive excess minerals and organic nutrients leading to the proliferation of plant material, especially algae. This in turn causes a reduction in the dissolved oxygen content in the water which leads to the extinction of other aquatic organisms.

There have been changes on the lake and its surroundings. Its hydrology has certainly changed through water diversions in the upper watershed areas, for the purpose of irrigating agricultural developments. On the other end, a dam was constructed in 1921 at the outlet into the Link River. Lake flushing flows - essential for nutrient export - have been altered and the level of the water in the lake has been lowered below the levels prior to 1921. Lowered water levels contribute to the increased winds that cause disturbance of the shallow waters. That agitation induces re-suspensions of the sediment at the bottom of the lake. Altogether, these factors cause hypereutrophication that further stimulate algae growth. In essence, if one were to set about designing a habitat for algae, this would be an ideal setting. Nature performed that job with utmost distinction.

As you recall, the star player in this book drama is this very Aphanizomenon flos-aquae (AFA). It has become, the most dominant micro-algae (read again, cyanobacteria) among the phytoplankton in Upper Klamath Lake. This is the normal pattern, at least from about June to October each year. By the 1930's, the word to use then was 'abundant' (not yet 'dominant') but by the mid 1950's – make no mistake about it – AFA was the truly 'dominant' species on the lake. These blue-green algae form large colonies that resemble grass clippings from your summer lawn. They appear throughout the lake in late spring and continue to increase in density as high as 30,000 filaments per ml (that's really high!) by late summer. They rise, but then they fall. By early autumn, most of the AFA die naturally. Unfortunately, the decomposition of this large amount of biomass then creates undesirable conditions such as the depletion of dissolved oxygen and strong unpleasant odors. For this reason alone, **harvesting of the algae before it decomposes, is therefore ecologically useful and expedient.**

Careful observation has shown that the timing of the annual bloom correlates (not surprisingly) with the flow of the Williamson River. That river you recall originates from springs and collects runoff all through the humus-rich Klamath marsh and that tails off at the end of each summer. During dry years the flow ceases earlier than during wet years. And so, guess what? The AFA in the lake follows that same pattern.

The density of the AFA is not spread uniformly across the lake. A few bays have higher densities. The winds tend to concentrate the algae down wind and marshy areas tend to have lower concentrations. Samples taken from the deeper parts of the lake also show lower densities of all phytoplankton including AFA, but in other areas the AFA is so abundant at full bloom that it forms a thick mat on the surface of the water.

Whereas AFA dominates in the late spring and summer, at other times different species of algae are more abundant. The lake is also home to others like *Cryptomonas erosa* and in the early spring you see *Fragilaria* or *Stephanodiscus astrea*, among others. Lesser amounts of *Microcystis areuginosa* and *Coelospherium* often appear in July and these can sometimes persist into late Fall.

Despite possible competition from some of these other algae species, AFA does remain the dominant species from late May up to October or November, producing a biomass that can exceed 50mg per liter (that's again very high!). The blooms are often witnessed in two phases, with a first peak in late June to early July, and a second peak in late September to mid-October. Standing crop estimates have set the usual AFA dominated biomass on the lake at about 30 million kilograms at its peak.

The *Aphanizomenon flos-aquae* species is unique among the microalgae of the lake in its ability to fix nitrogen. That's a big plus, for it means that this cyanobacteria can take the nitrogen from the air and utilize it to make amino acids, (and hence proteins), directly. That allows it to choke the competition from other potential blooms during the active harvest season to favor its complete dominance in the biomass.

It's as if the AFA is on a mission. It knows its true destiny and therefore fights relentlessly to accomplish that. Nature cooperates beautifully by wiping out the competition and then declares victory. Typically, the lake sees about 300 days of sunlight each year, providing a near perfect growing environment for the AFA. Add to that the euphoric condition (with reduced levels of oxygen) and alkalinity of the water (high pH). These all favor the proliferation of the AFA bloom. The absence of heavy metals, pesticides, herbicides, insecticides, and fungicides only makes this expansive lake a most convenient habitat for growing what is shaping up to be a very important dietary supplement.

There is such an abundance of nutrients and organic matter flowing into the lake and being trapped there, that phytoplankton is not the only evidence of life forms. There is also an over abundance of midges and dense beds of larger aquatic weeds (macro-algae or macrophytes). The midge larvae (mainly *Chironomus*) grow in sediments at the bottom of the lake where the water is shallow (and that's most of the lake). Then as they mature, they rise to the surface in swarms often becoming somewhat of a nuisance (at least to boaters and really to anyone else coming near the lake). The shallow areas like Pelican Bay often get covered over with these 'aquatic weeds' (especially *Potarnogeton crispus*) and therefore do not attract those tourists or visitors intent on either sightseeing or recreation.

HARVESTING 'GOLDEN SCUM'

None of this is really new. For decades, Upper Klamath Lake has provided a remarkably stable abundance and highly available biomass of the *Aphanizomenon flos-aquae*. This effectively unlimited supply has provided the basis for a viable commercial industry, harvesting the blue-green algae for use as an important dietary supplement. From about 1980, a small number of commercial operators have been taking advantage of the opportunity. However, since this species of cyanobacteria is not conveniently cultured like *Spirulina* in outdoor ponds or raceways, it requires very different procedures for harvesting and processing. In the early days, there were two main harvesting methods[1].

The principal one at that time removed the AFA after it passed out of the lake into an irrigation canal at the south end of the lake (called the A-canal). From the canal a large series of screens was used to remove the biomass at the site of an abandoned low-head hydroelectric turbine facility, where there was a convenient 10-ft drop to allow a gravity feed. To first remove debris (including flotsam and some small amount of fish) at the head of the facility, they used front and rear nylon filter screens, which ranged from about 1.5 to 3 inches in mesh size along the front. The screens were placed in vertical slots in front of the inflows at the harvest facility. These screens clog with debris fairly quickly and so they had to be alternately lifted and manually cleaned from the back with pressured water. Further down, other nylon screens were used to filter the algae either using the elevation drop to disperse or pump the water over the screens. The collected biomass was sprayed with water to transfer it to a secondary vibrating filter screen to remove most of the unwanted material. Some of that would be made up of small crustaceans (like *Daphnia*) which are still used commercially as a food product for the aquaculture industry.

After passing through these vibrating screens, there would be a sludge of algae containing about o.1% solids. This would be pumped to a series of three slow-speed horizontal centrifuges, which then removed other small extraneous material. Interestingly enough, AFA has a specific gravity equal to water, allowing for the centrifugal separation of sand, silt and any other light filth.

The algae concentrate was then fed by gravity into a processing plant where a vertical centrifuge with high G-force application was used to separate cells and colonies, removing about 90% of the remaining water. At that stage, the algae product was about 6-7% solids. Once concentrated, the product was chilled to 2° C and stored before being pumped to freezers.

Turning back to the early AFA harvesting methods on the lake, there were other operators who did their collections on the open lake. They used self-powered barges with rotating screens to filter the AFA. One type of barge had rotating screens that were lowered just below the surface of the lake. Another type pumped the water plus biomass from underneath the surface to screens set up on the barge. Most of the algae typically float within a few feet of the surface, so those techniques made more product available than would be at greater depths. Usually, the product harvested in this manner was held on the barges at ambient temperatures or often it was chilled to about 4 degrees Celsius until the biomass could be ferried to a processing plant on shore.

All these conventional methods just described are essentially non-selective in extracting material from the lake. When used to extract AFA, for example, quite often the biomass that is collected contains undesirable components along with the target algae. The harvesters would work efficiently if the product being collected was the only, or at least the overwhelmingly dominant biomass in the body of water where harvesting was taking place. However, this is usually not the case. Other algae species or zooplankton are typically present in the same region. Therefore, these conventional harvesting techniques often led to undesirable contaminants such as certain fish species which tended to quickly decay and contaminate the algae.

Those methods are now outdated. The state of the art methodology for harvesting AFA utilizes **new advanced technology** for which a patent was filed by Desert Lake Technologies Inc. (DLT) a few years ago[2]. DLT is far and away the premier harvester on the lake today. "The technology was best described in the DLT patent, although even further improvements have been made since then."

Today, well equipped barges go on to the lake at propitious times for careful selective extraction of the *AFA*. The extreme selectivity of this modern method exploits a physical characteristic rather unique to AFA among the associated algae species. It turns out that AFA is a filamentous microalgae resembling a supple blade of grass. Contrary to other algae species with more rigid shapes, the AFA tends to adhere to surfaces or wrap itself around structures, such as a wire. Building on this essential property, barges with rotating wires have been developed to selectively harvest AFA and leave behind other species of algae. In effect, **the harvested algae product using this technology is virtually pure AFA.**

The extraction apparatus used in this patented technology consists of a rotating monofilament (typically, nylon) which acts as the transport agent, wrapped alternately around two conveyor drums. The first upper conveyor drum (diameter about 6") is fixed in location and rotates mechanically (by electric motor) to frictionally drive the monofilament. The second and lower conveyor drum (diameter about 2.5") is usually an idle drum rotated both by the monofilament and by the water below (into which it dips) as the barge moves forward. Surprisingly, the smaller size of the submerged drum increases the rate (yield) of AFA extraction, since suspended algae in the immediate vicinity tend to bypass the larger submerged drums. This probably relates to the predicted diverging streamlines of flow, as water passes over the submerged drums. The design is such as to create a downstream wake, like a hydrofoil configured to reduce separation or wake turbulence aft of the hydrofoil when submerged. As the barge moves through the water (usually at about 2 knots) the monofilament causes the AFA to adhere to it and by rotation lifts the product out of the lake, and then deposits it into the barge.

Spacing of the parallel adjacent portions of the monofilament can be controlled to facilitate selective extraction. If the spacing is too close, lateral bridging of extracted material can occur leading to further extraction of undesirable materials. On the other hand, maintaining a close spacing between adjacent segments and/or windings can increase overall rates (yield) of the desired material extraction. Therefore, spacing is typically about half an inch between adjacent monofilaments but that can vary between 3/8" and 1".

Another variable would be the travel time of the extracted AFA on the monofilament which affects the extent to which water is eliminated in this first step. This allows an operator to at least partially time the rate of AFA extraction to a point where the liquid content in the initial product is compatible with secondary-processing parameters. The adjustment is made by varying the drive-speed at which the upper horizontal drum is rotated (by varying the motor speed). This determines the time AFA is on the monofilament between the water in the lake and the upper discharge end of the conveyor. That distance may also vary by raising or lowering the idle drum in the lake. Typically this first AFA extracted product contains about 1% to 2% solids.

When the AFA adhering to the monofilament reaches the top of the upper conveyor drum, a simple adjustable metal or plastic strip (with silicone rubber edge) acts as a scraper to remove the AFA from the monofilament. The AFA is then deposited, by falling under gravity onto a conveyor belt to maximize de-watering. The product is then typically 3-5% solids. It is afterward chilled by passing through a heat exchanger and finally collected into storage containers on the barge. These containers are usually also chilled and insulated to maintain the AFA at a temperature around 2°C (36°F) until it is removed for secondary processing. This chilling procedure is one of the most important factors in preserving the nutrient integrity of harvested algae. It generally takes just minutes from the AFA leaving the water to get into the refrigerated tanks, right there on each barge while harvesting takes place.

Of course, the 'fresh' portion of the monofilament is then continuously returned and that is again ready to interact with more AFA in the lake as it cycles back.

During the blooming AFA season (late May/June to late Oct/Nov), each day prior to harvesting, samples of algae are collected and ana- lyzed in a floating lake laboratory to ensure the quality and purity of the bloom. These biomass measurements include the quantity of algae per volume of water and species analysis. Once the purity (greater than 99%) of an algae bloom has been established, harvest- ing operations can begin.

As the barge gets into the harvesting zone determined from the observation of the exact location of the AFA and its apparent depth of distribution, an operator can then adjust the various parameters to optimize the yield. They would look for wind and water currents and make adjustments. The submersible lower drum can be let down to a depth of 6-8 feet below the water surface depending on the appar- ent depth of the highest AFA concentration. The innovative technol- ogy is well advanced today. Based on the experience of a few years, whenever the weather cooperates it has become routine to harvest fresh reliable, high-quality AFA. That harvested cyanobacteria is then on its way to becoming a standardized food supplement that is earning its place at the forefront of Stem Cell Nutrition.

But it still remains to be processed.

PROCESSING OF AFA

At the processing plants, the harvested AFA is treated by another proprietary process of centrifugation and filtration(3). This step is also designed to concentrate certain components, including specifi- cally, the *L-selectin blocker* responsible for supporting the release of stem cells from the bone marrow. Typically, this more concentrated AFA contains much more of the glycoprotein that we met in Chapter 5. It is enriched in this way by a factor of about five, compared to the fresh AFA coming directly from the lake.

The concentrate of AFA is then dried using a further proprietary process – a drying technology called Hydro Dri™. This is an innovative drying method that uses heat transfer and the specific properties of water to gently remove moisture from the AFA. The wet algae extract is progressively dispensed at one end, on to a moving food-grade Mylar conveyor belt (about 4-5 ft. wide), supported by computer-controlled hot water tables. Drying takes place by conduction as heat from the hot water supporting the belt is transferred to the water in the AFA extract which then evaporates. This leaves a thin film of dried flakes which are then collected at the other end.

For the curious reader, here's how that drying process works. Consider this. When water is placed over a heating source, infrared (heat) energy is transferred throughout the water by convection. The heat energy then *radiates* from the water, primarily through evaporation. Now, when water is covered by a transparent membrane like plastic and placed over a heating source the surface evaporation cannot take place. The major heat loss is blocked or refracted so that only *conductive* heat loss takes place. The plastic membrane acts like a mirror reflecting the infrared energy back into the water. So far, so good. Now let's go one step further. If a moist raw material (like the AFA extract above) is placed on the plastic membranes top surface, the water present therein creates a 'window' that allows for the passage of infrared energy through that moist material. The heat behaves as if there was no membrane in that location and is directly transferred to the water present in the material at the window. In just a few moments, the water in the material on the plastic membrane's surface evaporates and then the 'window' of infrared energy closes. That heat energy then 'refracts back' into the heated water sources, no longer exposing the material (the dry AFA in this use) to additional undesirable heat.

Here's the net result. As the AFA extract travels down on the Mylar conveyor, the water in it evaporates through the *'window'* in a matter of moments, with the 'window' closing in proportion to the rapid dissipation of water in the extract. Since Mylar itself is a poor heat conductor, once the AFA extract dries, the *'refractance window'* closes, and only a miniscule amount of heat is transferred to the product as it is carried to the end of conveyor system. **The AFA dried through the Hydro Dri™ system is exposed to heat for only a brief time, thereby delivering a dried product close to its natural state.**

This proprietary drying technology gently removes all residual water from the AFA extract, while maintaining integrity of all the nutrients and active compounds found in AFA. The superior efficiency of the method has been confirmed in an independent study performed at Washington State University.

The dried AFA product is then subjected to a series of stringent tests to confirm its safety and purity. It is then available for use as an ingredient in dietary food supplements. When appropriate, it is properly packaged, labeled and stored in modern refrigerated facilities.

For any edible product – be it any food or nutrition supplement – quality is key. In the next chapter, therefore, we go on to address issues of quality, safety and toxicity.

CHAPTER 9

Standards Of Excellence

In all matters pertaining to foods and drugs, quality assurance is always a central issue. Standards of excellence in this arena are not just desirable, they are indispensable. The consequences are huge, because the general public is always at risk. Therefore, the commitment must be absolute.

That's also true regarding the human consumption of AFA. All harvesters in the industry must have a sophisticated program to perform several sampling procedures and tests, throughout the harvesting and production process, to carefully monitor their product quality. Therefore, each batch of the biomass collected on a daily basis has to be rigorously documented, carefully sampled and adequately tested for key potential contaminants. That's a given.

QUALITY ASSURANCE

Routine quality control tests must monitor the algae coming from the lake for different classes of possible contaminants. These include cyanobacterial species *other than AFA*; any microorganisms (bacteria), heavy metals or pesticides; chlorophyll, moisture levels and perhaps most important of all, neurotoxins and hepatotoxins (especially microcystin).

It has been well documented that cyanobacteria, in general, can produce harmful toxins[1]. There are literature reports of other *Aphanizomenon* producing neurotoxins including saxitoxins (STX) and anatoxin -a. However, it is important to point out that **all tests on algae harvested from Klamath Lake (over 20 years) have failed to detect any significant cyanobacterial *neurotoxins*.** The only cyanotoxin found during that period of time was microcystin- a type of hepatotoxin- that appeared in samples of a different species of lake phtyoplankton known as *Mycrocystis*. Again, note that the incidence of microcystin – the toxin - only bears a correlation to the presence of *Mycrocystis* – the alga. **No confirmed reports have ever been documented of *Aphazinomenon flos-aquae* itself producing microcystin (*hepatotoxin*).**

Nevertheless, there are four different analytical methods (test assays) that have been used to detect and even quantify the various possible cyanotoxins:

i. Mouse Bioassay for the detection of neurotoxins (SFXs, anatoxin –a)

ii. Spectrophotometric Enzyme Assay for the presence of acetycholinesterase inhibiting neurotoxin (anatoxin-a)

iii. Enzyme- Linked Immunosorbant Assay (ELISA) for detection of microcystins.

iv. Protein Phosphatase Inhibition Assay (PPIA) for detection of microcystins.

Here's a typical routine. During the harvesting season, the dried AFA ends up in boxes that contain about 450 kg of frozen algae which are taken to the plant for quality testing and further processing. On different days, the yield may range anywhere from 20 – 300 or more boxes which must obviously be carefully labeled. A one kilogram sample is removed from each box. A statistical method called Acceptance Sampling is then used to determine the number of these samples from each batch that needs to be pulled for a composite sample to be representative of the complete batch in each case. Frozen composite samples are freeze dried, homogenized with a sifter and then analyzed. Batches are kept frozen until the test results are received. When a batch passes the tests, it is freeze-dried and then released for processing into the finished consumable product, such as capsules or tablets.

Quality is indeed a most important issue and a few additional observations are relevant here.

Screening for neurotoxins

Two strains of algae associated with *Aphanizomenon* have been reported to produce neurotoxins. The first is NH-5 which produces saxitoxins and that is definitely **not** the same species as *Aphanizomenon Flos-aquae*, found in Klamath Lake. The other is *Anabaena flos-aquae* which produces neurotoxins (both saxitoxins and anatoxins). This latter strain does occur in small amounts in Klamath Lake early in the season, and prior to the start of harvesting AFA. Therefore, to make assurance doubly sure (as Shakespeare would say) it is obviously prudent to screen the AFA product for these potentially harmful neurotoxins. The AOAC (Association of Official Analytical Chemists) *Mouse Bioassay* is now routinely used to screen test for these neurotoxins (STYs and anatoxin –a) in the algae harvested from Klamath Lake. This method is typically used for detecting STXs in shell fish but it is adapted here for algae in the absence of a standard method. The limit of detection for STXs with this method is 3 micrograms per gm of dried algae. In the case of shellfish, the quarantine limit for that STX to become a concern for human consumption is 80 micrograms per 100 gm meat. This assumes a typical meal might include about 100 gm of shellfish, equivalent therefore to 80 micrograms of STX. In the case of the algae, one would have to consume at least 27 gm at once (possibly close to 100 common capsules) if it contained no more than 3 micrograms per gm to attain this working threshold[2]. This is the worst case scenario of maximum concentration defining minimum consumption for there to be any harmful effect. The lethal dose is about 6-13 times higher. So there is no reason for STX to be a concern, once the screening with the AOAC Mouse Bioassay proves negative for each batch of AFA.

The situation with anatoxin-a is even more reassuring. The limit of detection for anatoxin-a by the same (AOAC) assay is 5 micrograms per gm of dried algae. The lowest observed adverse effect level for this neurotoxin has been established at 100 micrograms per kilogram of body weight. A person would have to consume almost 1.4 kgm (!) of algae containing no less than 5 micrograms per gram (the limit of detection) to reach any toxic level. An alternative assay to monitor contamination by the toxic *Anabaena flos-aquae* uses a colorimetric determination of cholinesterase activity. It is based on the fact that anatoxin-a inhibits that enzyme. As if that were not enough, still another method has also been used to detect anatoxin –a, this time using high performance liquid chromatography (HPLC) and fluorescence detection.

Again, it is worth emphasizing that despite all the screening that has taken place over decades (and is still taking place), no cyanobacterial neurotoxins have been detected in the dried AFA harvested from Klamath Lake, when examined by either the AOAC mouse bioassay or HPLC- florescence detection. There is no reasson for concern here.

Screening for hepatotoxins

The cyanobacterial populations found in Klamath Lake can have two possibly dangerous components. These are *Microcystis* and *Oscillatoria*, both of which are known to produce the hepatotoxins known as microcystins. If microcystins are ingested in significant concentrations, the consequences could be very serious. It could lead to acute liver damage and in the extreme, to death.

Two methods are used to determine the possible content and activity of these microcystins. The first is the ELISA immunoassay, a method to determine just the possible content of hepatotoxins. It is based on polyclonal antibody, developed by Chu et al. over twenty years ago[3]. However, not all microcystins (even when present) are actually bioactive. Therefore, to determine the actual toxic effect, a second method is used which is based on the fact that microcystins are specific potent inhibitors of some protein phosphatse enzymes. This so-called PPIA assay measures that inhibition which correlates with the toxins' ability to promote tumors and to provoke liver damage[4]. The assay is 1000 times more sensitive than the mouse bioassay or the HPLC – fluorescence assay[2].

When the microcystin levels that have been detected were compared with phytoplankton composition of biomass samples from Klamath Lake, it was pretty obvious that the microcystin was being produced by the Microcystis species. **To be more specific, there have been no confirmed reports ever of microcystin being produced by** *Aphanizomenon flos-aquae* **in the lake.** Period.

The State of Oregon's Department of Agriculture (DOA) has set a safe limit of 1 microgram of microcystin per gram of dry weight of algae product. This level was based, not without some rationale, upon the guideline set by a World Health Organization panel for a safe acceptable level in drinking water. Assuming a person would drink up to 2 litres of water per day, the regulatory value was set at 1 microgram per litre of water. But the Oregon DOA did not define a standard method for monitoring microcystin content. The ELISA and PPIA assays correlate well but the ELISA method tends to overestimate the levels consistently and that's the one that is routinely used. However, it's always better to be safe than sorry.

Microcystin has indeed been the subject of unnecessary controversy in the past. It clearly introduces the question of safety with respect to consumption of any blue green algae from Upper Klamath Lake. It therefore deserves further consideration since that's taking this author back to medical school, almost 30 years ago.

SAFETY

Every medical student learns an ethical mantra, dubiously attributed to the original and famous Hippocratic Oath that doctors subscribe to, which simply says "above all, do no harm". This is a fundamental principle guiding every form of medical intervention and it must apply just as well for any unconventional use of botanical products, including algae and the cyanobacteria that we have focused on here – namely *Aphanizomenon flos-aquae*.

In practical terms, what the phrase implies is that when given an existing physical situation, it may be better not to do something, or even to just do nothing, than to risk causing more harm than good. In other words, all healthcare professionals and wise consumers alike, must continuously do what is called risk/benefit analysis regarding every choice that is made. Almost every intervention- be it a clinical procedure, use of a pharmaceutical preparation, or dietary supplement, any or other alternative/complementary therapy – will have associated risks and potential benefits. The two elements must always be considered and proportionally weighted. That is wisdom at its best.

Now, in the case of AFA, we have mentioned the basic assays that are used for quality assurance and referenced the most important potential contaminant – namely, the hepatotoxin, microcystin. To be more unnecessarily precise, microcystins are a family of several dozen different cyclic peptides that can indeed be very toxic to both plants and animals, including *homo sapiens*. If ever ingested, microcystin would travel to the liver through the biliary transport system, where it might tend to accumulate. It could bind to protein phosphatases (inhibiting those liver enzymes) and thereby interfere with cellular control processes. If so, this could potentially lead to serious problems. Therefore, this question of possible microcystin contamination of AFA demands the complete risk/benefit analysis just mentioned above.

What then is the real microcystin risk?

We may begin with the conclusion that after 30 years of AFA human consumption by many thousands, if not millions of consumers, **there has been no confirmed case of microcystin toxicity resulting from ingestion of any algae product derived from Klamath Lake**. However, the details are very important, so we must elucidate further.

Microcystin is not new and neither is the source from which it comes – namely, *Microcystis*, which has always been found as a minor constituent among the phytoplankton in Klamath Lake. This particular blue-green algae came into prominence specifically in 1996 because a substantial bloom was surprisingly observed that particular summer on the lake. Expert consultants were brought in. Dr. Wayne Carmichael from the Department of Biological Sciences at Wright State University in Dayton Ohio and Dr. Donald Anderson from the Biology Department, Woods Hole Oceanographic Institution in Massachusetts, reviewed the situation which was brought to the public's attention as well as to the Oregon Health Division (OHD), whose officials naturally became concerned for public safety.

At that time there were just a few proposed guidelines regarding microcystin, based on single studies which obviously had associated uncertainty. Therefore, an unrestricted grant was awarded to the University of Illinois to complete a comprehensive risk assessment. A review was undertaken of more than 300 related scientific publications in order to accurately evaluate the potential risk associated with microcystin as a possible contaminant of blue-green algae products. After completion of this risk assessment, it was proposed that a safe level of microcystin should be considered as 10 micrograms per gram of dried algae product. Furthermore, Dr. Gary Flamm (who was a former head toxicologist at the USFDA in Washington, DC) later performed a separate risk assessment and concluded a safe level for microcystin would be 5 micrograms per gram. This was the same level of safety supported by Dr. Carmichael in a written testimonial when he and his team did their safety review.

Nevertheless, the Oregon Health Division exercised more than an abundance of caution and passed a regulation that established 1microgram per gram as the maximum acceptable concentration of microcystin. To put that further in context, based on animal studies alone, the actual safe level of intake would be between 2500 and 6000 micrograms of microcystin per day. To widen the safety margin, this was reduced by a factor of 1000. In other words, the regulation calls for a safe level at 1microgram per gram that is about 1000 times lower than that established as safe in animal studies. Liver damage could be anticipated only at levels that exceed 10,000 times the adopted safe level. **A person would have to consume more than 5,000 normal capsules per day to attain those ridiculous levels.** It's all about actual concentration.

It should also be emphasized that the state-of-the-art harvesting method in use today specifically isolated AFA, as was explained in the last chapter. All the other quality assurance safeguards are now in place in the industry to validate the extremely high quality of AFA that is processed eventually into formulations that are convenient for human consumption. By being proactive and technically responsible, the industry has gained an excellent reputation over several years.

What's the bottom line here? **Microcystin could be definitely toxic to the liver in a different situation, but it is completely safe at any levels currently found in blue-green algae products that are routinely screened for this possible contaminant. With confirmed levels below the 1 microgram per gram standard, the absolute risk is practically ZERO!**

It is true that no one likes to even think of the word toxicity, much less to risk any possible exposure. But that we can't avoid. There are toxins virtually everywhere – in the air we breathe, in the food we eat and in the water we drink. We live in a world surrounded on every hand by potentially harmful microorganisms, poisonous natural products, heavy metals and other toxic chemicals. But we need not become paranoid, lest our anxiety become a bigger problem than the actual exposures we face almost daily. Again, it all comes down to real numbers – the actual concentrations of each potential toxin.

Still the facts speak for themselves. Food-borne illness and disease (typically, food poisoning) is widespread in America despite the best efforts of the authorities who conduct regular food inspection and who impose strict health regulations. Some food-borne illnesses arise from improper handling, preparation and storage of food, and the best precaution from a public health standpoint, is proper and regular hand washing. But much of it also arises from food contamination with natural chemicals, pesticides, additives, heavy metals and even medicines that get into the food supply.

Some of the most common bacterial pathogens include *Campylobacter jejuni, Clostridium perfringens, Salmonella spp., enterohemorrhagic E.coli* and, of course, the common E. coli that causes the frequent travellers' diarrhea. But there are many others and that's only the beginning. Think of all the viruses that cause one third of the cases of food poisoning in developed countries. Add the effect of food-borne parasites and we're still considering just the live microorganisms.

But then there are the mycotoxins like aflatoxins (from nuts and seeds, for example,) or *patulin* (from fruits), or *tricothecenes* (from maize, wheat, corn or rice) and the long list goes on. Several foods (usually plants) can contain toxins naturally. They produce them perhaps as their desperate line of defense for their own survival. They cannot run away like animals do in their fight for survival. So they produce poisonous alkaloids and other natural products to kill off their 'prey.'

We could go on to lament the presence of *pesticides* that show up in many agricultural foods, and then there are the heavy metals (like mercury and lead) that show up sometimes in fish. Many studies confirm the nature of these problems not only for domestic food suppliers but even more so for some imported foods, where standards leave much to be desired. But the more we focus on these issues and all the associated environmental factors, the more depressing this subject does become. The point is that **unwanted and unhealthy ingredients in the normal food supply are as ubiquitous as food itself.** The issue of possible effects from contamination by microcystin in cyanobacteria derived from Klamath Lake is neither unusual nor new. Relatively speaking, and in practical terms, it does become inconsequential. That's just the way it is.

The net effect of all that food contamination is that each year in the United States, there are estimates of some 50 million cases of food-borne illnesses, leading to over 100,000 hospitalizations and more than 3,000 deaths[5]. This food contamination naturally creates an enormous social and economic strain in society. The estimated costs - both in medical costs and lost productivity – run into about $40 billion each year. So these issues are by no means insignificant.

Given all this and much more that could be said, it is obvious that the concern regarding food safety is generally not the existence or even the presence of toxins in food. That would be a qualitative issue. Far more importantly, it always relates to the quantitative aspect – that is, the actual concentration of any potential toxin or other contaminant. Then the question becomes relative to some established safety level. In practice therefore, **whenever a compound is found in any food at a concentration below the level that has been determined to be safe for that compound, then the food is considered to be safe, with respect to that compound.** Such is the case for AFA with respect to microcystin, and eminently so. **The absence of any confirmed case of toxicity arising from the consumption of these dietary supplements over decades perhaps makes the case better than anything else.**

TOXICITY

But that is clearly not enough. The US Food and Drug Administration, as well as international organizations like the Organization for Economic Cooperation and Development, require toxicological investigations before a product can be registered as 'Generally Recognized As Safe', (GRAS) for human consumption. This important GRAS designation demands that both short term and long term toxicity studies with rodents be done to demonstrate the product's safety. (Obviously, similar *human* studies would be rather unethical, to say the least).

Both sub-acute toxicity (up to 14 days) and sub-chronic toxicity (up to 90 days) of extracts of the AFA blue green algae have been studied in rats by independent researchers at the College of Veterinary Medicine, University of Illinois at Urbana[6,7].

In the sub-acute toxicity study, groups of 12 rats of each sex were given either 5% glycerin in water (controls) or 600 mg/kg of the AFA product prepared in 5% glycerin in water for two weeks by oral gavage. They were then observed for a further two weeks. The researchers found that the administration of AFA had no effect on behavior, food and water intake, growth or survival. There were no deficiencies between treated and control groups for all the important variables of hematology and clinical chemistry, when analyzed at the end of the dosing and observation periods. After the most sensitive and ethical sacrificing of the rodents, a careful post mortem examination was performed. Again, there was no significant difference observed in the many organs examined and the histopathology of different organs and tissues were indistinguishable between the treated and control animals. Sperm motility parameters were also similar for control and treated males.

The authors were compelled to conclude that 'the AFA extracts, when administered at doses about 20 times the maximum normally recommended daily dose, did not produce any adverse effects in the Wistar rats after sub-acute treatment'[6].

In a follow-up study published the following year, the same research group reported the results of a sub-chronic toxicity study of the same AFA extract. The study design and protocols were similar but this time the rats were each given either 5% glycerin in water (controls) or 20 mg/kg of the AFA extract prepared in 5% glycerin in water for 90 days by oral gavage. The results again were almost identical for both the treated and control animals after this extended period. The researchers again concluded that 'the AFA extract, even at doses about 7 times the maximum normally recommended dose, did not produce any adverse effects in Wistar rats, after such sub-chronic treatment'[7].

No Tumor Growth

The evidence was clear and that would normally be enough for a food product or dietary supplement. But, unique to this particular dietary supplement is the fact that it does enhance bone marrow-derived stem cells (BMDSCs). Stem cells are pluripotent as we have seen and therefore, in principle, they can give rise to tumors if they proliferate and/or differentiate outside of normal control. Moreover, tumors appear to be able to attract peripheral blood stem cells that would tend to increase vascularity. Therefore BMDSCs may enhance the development of existing tumors by forming new blood vessels. In fact, the growth rate of a tumor is intimately linked to the development of new blood supply, which in turn could be enhanced by circulating BMDSCs. It was already demonstrated that incorporation of endothelial precursor cells into the blood vasculature of a tumor correlates with the tumor growth.

Now then, if circulating stem cells were to contribute to tumor vasculature and hence to tumor growth, when you increase the number of circulating stem cells, such as by AFA consumption, that might by itself accelerate tumor growth. So the question does arise, could this AFA consumption lead to increased tumor formation or growth?

This question has been recently addressed, at least in one study out of the Department of Veterinary Biosciences, University of Illinois at Urbana and the AntiCancer Inc. laboratories in San Diego, California. Researchers applied principles and procedures outlined in the NIH Guide for the Care and Use of Laboratory Animals to produce an orthotopic model of human breast cancer in mice[8]. Some mice were assigned equally to treated (experimental) or control groups. All the mice were surgically transplanted with human

MDA-MB-435-GP breast cancer directly into their mammary fat pads. For the experimental group, each of the animals was then gavaged daily for 6 weeks with 300 mg/kg of the AFA extract dissolved in phosphate-buttered saline (PBS). The control animals were similarly gavaged with PBS alone. The tumor growth was monitored using live whole body fluorescence imaging. At the end of the study, the tumors were excised and weighed.

What was the difference observed?

There was a surprise. At the start of the feeding trial, tumor areas for both the control and experimental groups were statistically identical. However, the tumor growth rate turned out to be **slower** in the animals fed with the AFA extract when compared to the control group. After 6 weeks, tumor areas were 40% larger in the control group and the tumor weight was 35% smaller in the treated group. In other words, feeding the animals with the AFA did **not** promote tumor growth but rather **reduced** the growth of human MDA-MB-435 breast cancer in this study.

The authors were tempted to speculate about the possible reason for this observed reduction in tumor growth. They suggested three possibilities. First, it is possible that after migrating into cancerous tissue, attracted by cytokines, and after proliferating and differentiating into cells of the target tissue, stem cells could secrete signals inhibiting cellular division.

Secondly, the AFA extract is a concentrate that contains the photosynthetic blue pigment phycocyanin that has been shown to have significant antioxidant and anti-inflammatory properties and even possible anticancer properties[9]. The third possibility might be the polysaccharide in AFA that was shown to stimulate Natural Killer (NK) cell activity and support NK cell migration[10]. NK cells could inhibit the tumor growth.

Whatever the possible mechanism here, the fact remains that the AFA extract - instead of promoting tumor growth - actually inhibited tumor growth, at least in this singular case. That's called 'going in the right direction', at least.

Speaking of direction --- there's a new direction emerging in industrialized societies. There is a growing momentum originally spearheaded by those younger baby boomers who were part of the loose association sometimes denoted as the Wellness Movement. Thanks to AFA and to Stem Cell Nutrition, the whole wellness concept itself is undergoing a Transformation. That's the focus of **Part Four** -the final section of this book. Let's briefly summarize where we are just before we move there.

12-Point
SUMMARY OF PART THREE

1. Intrinsic to nature is the supply of all the essentials for normal human life. Not all the natural sources present themselves with attractive colors and delightful tastes to make for a satisfying and sensual experience. Some are just plain and ordinary offerings that justify consumption in the end, if not at the beginning. Algae is among them.

2. Stem Cell Nutrition – with ordinary but specific algae presently at center stage – appeared naturally and spontaneously, more by unintended default than by human craftiness.

3. For hundreds of years, several species of algae have been used as food in different parts of the world and in some cases, they have been associated with forms of traditional medical treatment. AFA is a modern dietary innovation.

4. Edible seaweeds (macroalgae) have gained widespread acceptance, particularly in Southeast Asia. Three of the most common types are Porphyra, Laminaria and Undaria pinnatifida.

5. More recently, the microalgae (including cyanobacteria) have gained fairly widespread acceptance. They are known as much for their reported benefits to health as for their value as food ingredients. The three dominant players in this area are Spirulina, Chlorella and Aphanizomenon flos-aquae (AFA).

6. AFA blooms annually (May—October) in almost unlimited abundance in Upper Klamath Lake, Oregon. This lake is one of the largest freshwater lakes in the US and it receives a steady inflow of nutrients from the surrounding marshes and springs.

The pristine environment, with convenient rainfall and copious sunlight provides idyllic habitat for AFA to thrive.

7. Modern technology has made it possible to harvest the AFA in season very selectively. The product is initially concentrated on site and chilled to retain quality before it is stored and transported to plants on shore.

8. Patented technology using centrifugations and filtration, allows for specific concentration of the L-selectin blocker, a crucial ingredient in AFA.

9. An innovative drying method uses heat transfer and the specific properties of water to gently remove moisture from the AFA concentrate. This leaves a thin film of dried flakes for final processing into tablets/capsules as necessary for diet supplementation.

10. Batches of AFA harvested from Upper Klamath Lake are routinely monitored for quality. Tests included in the protocols screen for other contaminating species, hepatotoxins, (especially microcystin), microorganisms, heavy meals, pesticides and more.

11. Microcystin is toxic to the liver but it is completely safe at all levels currently found in all the blue-green algae products that are routinely screened for this possible contaminant.

12. The absence of any confirmed case of toxicity, arising from the consumption of these blue-green algae products after such widespread use over decades, makes the case – unambiguously - for extreme quality and safety. Both acute and chronic toxicity studies in animals have only confirmed that.

Stem Cell Nutrition promises to transform both the understanding and the application of wellness principles in the coming years. Therefore, in Chapter 10 that follows next, we draw stark contrasts between **Stem Cell Nutrition** and *Stem Cell Medicine* to make the case for wellness as the appropriate approach to life and health today. Then in Chapter 11, we attempt to describe *A Wellness Lifestyle* that incorporates a number of factors that impact health and stem cells, in particular. Finally, we formally conclude the book with mere speculation on *The Stem Cell Future*, for what that's worth. However, the fact that Stem Cell Nutrition offers a practical solution for a mild but significant enhancement of the normal renewal system of the body makes that intervention eminently reasonable.

Part 1V

The Wellness Transformation

transformation: *the act or process of becoming something new and different; a change in content or character; assuming a new nature or state.*

Preamble to Part Four

Throughout this book, we have referred fairly consistently to 'optimizing wellness' or 'optimizing health', where these somewhat interchangeable terms have been used in the broadest and most general sense, without definition or explanation. That was deliberately deferred for this final part of the book where it will actually now become the focus.

The concept of wellness, especially in the context of alternative medicine has been traced back to the 1950s when Halbert Dunn, MD first coined the phrase 'High level Wellness'. He delivered a series of lectures at a church in Arlington, Virginia, in which he defined his new phrase as *"an integrated method of functioning which is oriented toward maximizing the potential of which the individual is capable. It requires that the individual maintain a continuum of balance and purposeful direction within the environment where he is functioning."* More simply perhaps, he described wellness as "a direction in progress toward an even higher potential of functioning."

However, the concept did not give rise to a growing movement and then to a culture shift, until some twenty years later. By the 1970's, several trends were coming together. There was a growing reaction to the impact of technology on the food and nutrition industry. There was somewhat of a disillusionment with the medical establishment because the practice of medicine had become more and more high-tech, with all kinds of new diagnostics, invasive surgical procedures, and a host of new drugs and therapies for maintaining life and limb. Despite all this, there was still persistence of major chronic diseases and clearly an epidemic of illnesses resulting from poor lifestyle choices. Then there was the focus on 'back to basics' with a new reverence for the environment and all things natural, including food.

Finally, include a wave of some form of 'new spirituality with its celebration of life and an emphasis on harmony of body, mind and spirit. Put it all together, and the 'wellness philosophy' emerged and spread across Western culture, to gain increasing acceptance.

Now there was something more to aspire to, beyond the freedom from clinical illness and disease. Baby boomers wanted to preserve their youth and vitality indefinitely. Their new passion for health and fitness was giving the Wellness Movement a new momentum that increasingly impacted the culture in a variety of ways. The media became enchanted by a new class of 'gurus' and 'wellness advocates and practitioners.' These self-styled professionals and pioneers wrote runaway bestsellers and dominated ever-popular talk shows on television to advance their cause. Wellness was being promoted as a 'way of life', a new 'awareness' and the ultimate in 'self-actualization'. It became a holistic philosophy that sought to do justice first to the individual in a quest for actualization, them to a village in search of community and even to a planet in need of preservation.

There was only a loose association of those individuals embracing this Wellness Movement of the 70's and '80's, but it was a movement nonetheless. It made the shift to natural foods and the use of dietary supplements acceptable to a significant subset in the culture. It popularized fitness clubs and alternative therapies. It even glamorized the practice of meditation and a kind of New Age consciousness that denied all empiricism. Put it all together, and here was a new generation of 'wellness' disciples, drawn together with different convictions and personal agendas but all committed to experiencing the potential of life at their individual best. The wellness paradigm had arrived.

Whatever else the Wellness Movement did at the turn of the last century, at least it underscored four important principles that needed to invade the contemporary health scene. These principles began to help transform the culture and make the best of health attainable, especially in affluent industrial societies.

The first wellness focus was on *personal responsibility*. As the capability of doctors and other healthcare providers advanced by leaps and bounds, there had been a tendency to leave the onus of 'healthcare' to those who dispense 'medical care.' Judging from all the sensational news headlines, there could have been a tendency to neglect one's responsibility for 'self-care', with the misguided presumption that whatever went wrong could be readily restored by a visit to the family doctor or local clinic. If things really got bad, then a short stay in hospital would summon the best of medical care to one's disposal and all could be restored. There was a wonder drug for every conceivable condition and when that failed, modern surgical techniques could restore structure and function to any body part or else, the last resort could be organ transplantation.

But no, that was a self-defeating paradigm. **Doctors could never do for patients what only patients should do for themselves.** In the final analysis, it's what one does between their medical visits that truly determines health outcomes. The quality of health we enjoy would reflect the cumulative effect of all the daily lifestyle choices we make. There is no substitute for avoiding all the negative health influences like smoking, drug and alcohol abuse, lack of exercise with sedentary habits, poor sleeping routines, junk food diets, risky sexual behavior, dangerous and careless driving, constant negative attitudes or poor stress management. Even compliance with good medical advice requires the patient's cooperation. Doctors cannot and should not even attempt to live their patient's lives. There are clear boundaries for assistance and counsel, and then the patient must assume personal responsibility.

The concept of wellness does encourage exactly that. The experience of the best of health – including its promotion, maintenance and expansion - must begin with the individual awareness and a sense of personal responsibility that leads to the best lifestyle choices. Yes, **we do become what we eat, but also much more than that. Good lifestyle choices will favor good health consequences.** There is just no substitute for that. The Wellness Movement certainly encouraged that shift.

The second focus that proved to be very effective was the renewed emphasis on *prevention* rather than cure. That was the title for the most popular magazine publication that regularly advocated wellness by its consistent message, if not by an articulated mission. No one should deny that the prevention of illness is the ultimate solution to any health crisis we could face. It's the best approach for the individual committed to both quality of life and length of life. It's the best economic strategy for any public policy aiming to reduce the runaway costs of health care. And, in the final analysis, it's the moral imperative of all stakeholders in the industry.

Medicine is exceptional in delivering acute emergency care in crisis. The daily heroics that take place inside any emergency ward provide compelling testimony to that fact. Medicine is also very good in delivering relief to chronic symptoms and reducing morbidity when patients must unfortunately live with incurable disease. Even at the end of life, medicine delivers compassionate, palliative care that relieves suffering and pain and allows for 'death with dignity.'

But all this sophisticated resource that surpasses expectations and sometimes even imaginings, is delivered at the bottom of the heath cliff *after* patients have tumbled over the edge, for one reason or another. The professionals providing this excellent care at the bottom tend to resuscitate, stabilize, treat and restore many of these patients, who then get tossed back up on top the cliff, only to return back to medical centers as they continue to tumble over the unprotected edge.

The wellness crusade was a call for a renewed emphasis on prevention – a cry for the establishment of new guardrails along the edges of the health cliff everywhere. There certainly is a leadership role for good public health policy, but each rail could and should be erected one person at a time. Medical science and technology have made their greatest impact on humanity whenever a major advance was made on this front. Just think of the consequences derived from improved sanitation, the safety of the drinking water supply, regular hand washing, better housing, the development and use of vaccines, and so on. These types of preventive measures saved millions of lives. But then, as we celebrated the successes of modern medicine and the affluence of western culture, far too many of us presumed that medical care would be the answer to our negligence and stupidity. The more we celebrated the successes of recovery and cure, the less vigilant we became about health.

Thanks to the Wellness Movement (as nebulous as this really is, since no formal organization provides leadership or control) the culture has been pulling back. Nowhere is this more clearly seen than in attitudes to cigarette smoking. Today, it is bad economics – an excessive drain on the health care budget that is now showing signs of slowing down. But smoking has also become unsociable and even obnoxious to communities at large. Why should any society just continue to herald the efficacy of respiratory drugs and cardiac procedures, while we could promote, finance and defend smoking cessation programs? Why should the individual rely on professionals to cure heart and lung disease and insurance to finance the costs, rather than doing the responsible thing by butting-out before the consequences are manifest?

In every area of health, prevention is the preferred alternative. The responsible individual is thinking on a daily basis of all the lifestyle factors that are likely to reduce the role of disease. Wellness dictates that this must be almost an obsession, for it's clearly the best answer for anyone committed to engaging the highest quality of life anywhere.

A third focus that this so-called Wellness Movement re-emphasized was the tendency to search out *natural alternatives*. The widespread invasion of science and technology into every area of our modern lives has not been without some negative (perhaps unintended) consequences. Wellness advocates tended to presume that nature was intrinsically good and favorable to mankind. Technology was perceived in many instances, as introducing solutions to problems, while at the same time, introducing other problems. This is true in the physical environment, but it is also true as it pertains to health. Wellness considerations put the spotlight on things like additives in our food, municipal water contamination, air pollution, side effects of drugs, medical malpractice and iatrogenic illness. Obviously, there was a shift. A mistrust of applied science and technology developed, especially where health was concerned, and especially when illness or disease was not apparent. The search for alternatives led to the re-emergence of traditional and alternative therapies of many types and descriptions. Some proved to be more credible than others and gained increasing acceptance.

This led to a resurgence of 'health foods', 'natural foods' and 'organic foods'. In addition, there was increasing and widespread use of dietary supplementation to compensate for all the deficiencies of the industrialized food supply. There was an active search for all the traditional uses of all-natural products, including herbal remedies. Plus, a renewed emphasis on physical fitness made things like fitness centers, TV workouts and a number of programs designed to get the population moving again, all become as popular as ever. Several Eastern practices found a new acceptance in the West, including things like meditation and yoga, hypnosis, acupuncture, massage therapy and much more. The emphasis was on the natural non-invasive character of all these 'wellness activities", in contrast to the artificial aspects of modern medical science and technology.

A fourth and final principle underscored by the 'wellness approach' to health was the emphasis on *personal integration*. As modern medicine became more specialized, there was increasing tendency to neglect the whole person. Thus, the body was examined and treated as a collection of functioning parts. Each part was explored in sub-microscopic detail, with the inherent risk of 'missing the forest for the trees' (if we could mix metaphors). Wellness was moving in the opposite direction. Each individual is a unit. The body is an integral whole and health necessarily implies the harmonious functioning of all these collective parts. Moreover, the total person is comprised of body, mind and spirit and the health of each of these impacts the others, so that wellness could only be experienced as all aspects of health were simultaneously addressed. **There is a synergy to health that, by design, is indispensable to wellness in the twenty first century.**

Now then, over the past few decades, the spontaneous and unorganized social phenomenon that has been called the Wellness Movement has begun a transformation of healthcare, at least in North America. Millions of people have become increasingly aware and therefore have elected to pursue a new approach to their own health and well-being.

These wellness pioneers have first *taken responsibility* for their daily lifestyle, making choices and adopting habits that promote health and seek to *prevent* illness and disease. They have sought out the *natural alternatives* that they consider beneficial to optimizing their quality of individual life as a *whole person*. They are committed to experiencing the best of life for as long as possible, and to resort to 'allopathic restoration' only when all else fails and despite their best efforts.

If the pursuit of wellness has initiated a transformation of healthcare in recent times, then Stem Cell Nutrition now provides a new opportunity to make a further transformation of this phenomenon. The natural healing and renewal system of the body involves the spontaneous release of stem cells from the bone marrow and their role in repairing and restoring tissues and organs in the body. This recent discovery leads to a new understanding of how health is maintained from the inside, on a daily basis. It was an even more surprising discovery that a natural intervention like Stem Cell Nutrition can enhance this normal renewal process in a relatively mild but safe and significant way. **Stem Cell Nutrition therefore offers new possibilities for taking *responsibility* to practice *prevention*, and in a most natural way, it can influence the overall health of the *whole person*.** That is an opportunity for wellness transformation indeed.

In this final section of the book, we will explore these wellness ideas in more detail. We will compare and contrast the relationship of Nutrition and Medicine in Chapter 10, to underscore the proper role for **Stem Cell Nutrition**, in particular. In Chapter 11 we will consider the impact of different lifestyle factors, in order to examine what a **Stem Cell Lifestyle** might look like, and in Chapter 12 we will speculate on the possibilities of a **Stem Cell Future**.

CHAPTER 10

Stem Cell Nutrition
and Medicine

In the Information Age, both the practice of medicine from the doctor's point of view and the experience of medicine from the patient's point of view have changed in dramatic ways. There was a time when doctors enjoyed an authority and status in any community because of their vast exclusive knowledge that was gained through many years of training and work experience. They provided answers to important health questions and made dramatic interventions to ease pain or relieve other distressing symptoms, to control chronic diseases and often to save life. Patients had such respect for this important and even indispensable human science (and sometimes pure art), that they showed due deference to healthcare providers. Doctor's prescriptions were as good as commands and patient compliance could be usually taken for granted. In the area of health (and more so, disease), the doctor was king and the patient was subject.

Today, the doctor-patient relationship is entirely different. With the easy access to information – even specific, detailed information – many patients are prone to consider prescriptions as 'educated suggestions' which they have a right to evaluate. Therefore, on any given day in any city or town in industrialized society, there are many patients 'surfing the net' in search of more information regarding their symptoms, their presumed diagnosis and the prescriptions and advice they have received from their 'healthcare provider(s)' and anyone else. Some of this information is consistently authoritative and credible, from good sources and based on the best scientific research and historical data. But not all the dogma and associated claims are reliable. There is indeed much misinformation disseminated freely in the e-universe, some of which could even be dangerous.

This has led to an uneasy tension and sometimes confrontation in many a doctor-patient relationship. When there is inadequate communication and lack of trust, the patient tends to become non-compliant and the doctor experiences unnecessary and understandable frustration. Mutual trust and respect – on both sides – are essential for a proper working doctor-patient relationship.

Of all the points of controversy around wellness and medicine, perhaps none is as common and as divisive as the impact of nutrition and the associated dietary manipulation and supplementation. Although the admonition of Hippocrates thousands of years ago, to *'let food be your medicine and medicine your food,'* was very wise and very practical, some have abused this injunction with inappropriate and sometimes self-destructive applications. The central importance of dietary intake can hardly be overstated. In simple terms, we become what we eat. And in the computer age, this would be best underscored with the common adage 'garbage in, garbage out'. That's true. But that should never justify the foolhardy approach that disregards regular, appropriate health maintenance examinations. It is usually unwise to ignore clear definitive diagnostic results or to neglect proven beneficial therapeutic interventions when necessary.

The only rational and sensible approach that could prove to be responsible in any health situation is the combined emphasis on nutrition *and* medicine. One should always think and act holistically with the clear purpose of exploiting both of these resources simultaneously. Therefore, two questions must be asked. 'What natural, edible food or food product can I consume to help optimize my experience of health and wellness, now and in the future?' That's the first question. The second one is 'How can I apply the best medical intervention or therapy, based on proven science, to relieve my symptoms, if any, and improve my physical condition, now and in the future?' Answers to *both* of these questions become relevant to the experience of optimum health and wellness for everybody, everywhere, every day.

That is a fundamental approach worth emphasizing again and again. **'Nutrition *and* Medicine' is the only responsible and practical way forward. That is the future of healthcare.**

But some have drawn a false dichotomy. The case for nutrition *versus* medicine could only be justified in the practice of *primary prevention.* This is independent of any illness or disease. Even in perfect health, nutrition is protective and defensive, building and maintaining optimum health. In other words, it is critically important that we all have a diet that supplies adequate amounts of all the essential nutrients. Traditionally, that would refer only to the limited number of nutrients, deficiency of which has led to well-characterized diseases. That would refer to the classic food categories of proteins, carbohydrates, essential fats, vitamins and minerals. In addition, it is also critically important to avoid as much as possible 'poisons in our food' which are so prevalent in fast, processed and convenience foods. Those are filled with empty calories, unhealthy fats, additives of all kinds and much more. Good wholesome nutrition is an essential key in primary prevention. **One should never disregard the importance of nutrition.**

On the other extreme – when acute illness raises its ugly head, the refrain must always be 'nutrition, but medicine also.' In other words, regardless of the quality and adequacy of nutritional intake, when illness strikes, medicine is the appropriate response. **Nutrition is vital at home, very important in the hospital but almost irrelevant in the emergency room.** There is no substitute for urgent medical care. Thank God for skilled physicians and other medical staff who daily attend to acutely-ill patients. They do so with such amazing efficiency that miraculous results are anticipated every day. If nutrition has a role in primary prevention, then medicine has an indisputable role as the primary response to acute illness.

So there are two extremes. Nutrition as medicine is appropriate for primary prevention, even when enjoying the best of health. Yet nutrition is never enough when there is acute illness. At that time, medicine is the only responsible alternative. In the middle of these two extremes where the vast majority of people live, there are the common systemic complaints of everyday existence. There are the intrinsic risk factors that predispose many to degenerative conditions and often, there are also the chronic illnesses with which some unfortunate individuals are necessarily compelled to live. In all these situations, the most responsible lifestyle choice is to exploit the best of nutritional intake, including dietary supplementation, and the best of medical care. As such, wisdom is justified of all her children.

That makes the case for nutrition in general. Now, here's the application for **Stem Cell (SC) Nutrition** in particular. SC Nutrition is clearly a wise lifestyle choice as a form of primary prevention. This implies that even in the best of health, one might still seek to increase the number of circulating stem cells by the simple addition of proven AFA-derived products to a good balanced diet. Any other natural stem cell enhancer would make sense too. In the normal daily process of tissue cell renewal, the availability of stem cells in the circulation that can traffic to any specific tissues in need at any specific time can only enhance that renewal process. Therein is a significant component to building and maintaining optimum health which after all, is the essence of *primary prevention.*

In the second category we described above, when there are either obvious common complaints, indicative of tissue malfunction in some way, or when chronic illness is already present, or even the risk is increased for whatever reason, then SC Nutrition has a definite supportive role to play. This is true in the relief of symptoms, as malfunctioning and worn out tissues are constantly renewed by the trafficking of more stem cells from the bone marrow to the specific tissue sites involved. The application may be non-specific but it exploits all the potential benefits that nature normally pursues. SC Nutrition then becomes a natural intervention to alleviate symptoms and to help restore health and wellness. In a sense, this is *secondary prevention* at work, naturally.

In the more serious cases of acute illness or severe chronic conditions, SC Nutrition has obvious limitations and one must resort, in hope, to potential breakthroughs in **Stem Cell (SC) Medicine**. For example, in the case of acute myocardial infarction (or heart attack), there is now active research going on in several major medical centers to exploit the ability of stem cells injected into the circulation or directly into heart tissue soon after the event. This is with the intention of regenerating heart muscle and blood vessels to improve cardiac function and prognosis. Much progress is already being made. Other examples of this type of research were already mentioned back in Part 1, when we discussed 'exploiting the potential value of adult stem cells.' Many more are included in the Appendix at the back of the book. Stem Cells do offer the prospect of *regenerative medicine* which is the ultimate application of *tertiary prevention.* That is the best hope today for those who might suffer from serious chronic degenerative conditions. It is the research domain of SC Medicine.

In the event of acute illness, all the standard emergency room procedures and interventions remain the appropriate treatments of choice.

This is not the domain of SC Nutrition by any means.

All that aside, it is still useful and convenient here to make a direct comparison and draw a definite contrast between the approaches of Nutrition and Medicine, with respect to exploiting the unique characteristics of stem cells. We begin with their origins.

Origins of Nutrition and Medicine

Nutrition is as old as life itself. It is an indispensable characteristic of all living things. They all consume raw materials and by a normal process of metabolism, they convert that intake to maintain life and facilitate growth and repair. This has been the **life experience** from the beginning.

However, medicine as it refers to human intervention to alleviate illness and disease first began some 5,000 years ago with the ancient Egyptians. Yet for thousands of years, traditional medicine was more art than science and progress was very slow in coming. Perhaps the biggest quantum leap forward came with early advances in technology and agriculture that transformed public health and nutrition in the 19th century. This led to dramatic decline of the most lethal diseases. However, it is hard to imagine that the existence of microorganisms (germs) was discovered only in the 19th century and the production of antibiotics came about less than a hundred years ago. The application of the scientific method to medical research (as well as the concurrent advances in basic science and technology) revolutionized the practice of medicine in the 20th century. **Modern medicine definitely ranks among the pinnacles of all human achievement.**

Stem Cell Nutrition is a recent discovery of what essentially is an ancient phenomenon. In the first place, the normal tissue renewal process based on stem cells continuously released from bone marrow, is itself an intrinsic phenomenon that has just recently been brought to light. The first nutritional intervention that blocks L-selectin derives from the consumption of an ancient cyanobacteria that has been used traditionally as a dietary supplement, providing anecdotal benefits to health. Now our contemporary scientific understanding has caught up with nature's ordinary provision. *Homo sapiens are the winners.*

In contrast to this relatively easy and productive development in SC Nutrition, the implications and applications of SC Medicine have not kept pace. The latter is more like biotechnology, not biology. It is a human innovation, not a common natural phenomenon. Therefore, patience and persistence is necessary while active research proceeds around the world. Challenges have to be overcome, problems need to be solved and new discoveries have to be made. The origins of SC Medicine still remain somewhat obscure and elusive. But necessity remains 'the mother of all invention', so progress is being made. Hope for a major breakthrough abounds in many areas.

Discovery or Invention

Speaking of invention, it is worthy of note that SC Nutrition is truly not an invention. It is primarily and essentially just a discovery. It's simply the nature of things as they are and could be. As we pointed out before – **everybody has stem cells; everybody uses stem cells; everybody uses stem cells every day; stem cells work and ... they work every time.** This simple mantra underscores the natural, spontaneous and universal renewal process whereby stem cells leave the bone marrow, move in the peripheral circulation to tissues in need, whereupon they migrate to specific loci to proliferate and differentiate into cells of that particular tissue. Then we found out that this process could be enhanced by consuming normally occurring, edible natural product like microalgae (cyanobacteria) on a regular basis. That's the simplicity of SC Nutrition.

But there's nothing new happening here. What is new is our aware-ness and understanding of what nature does without much help from our creative minds or intriguing experimentation. There are no real problems to be solved or hurdles to be overcome in order to derive some new molecular phenomenon that is more a product of human ingenuity than of nature's spontaneity. We are therefore amazed by nature and not by our mental prowess.

SC Medicine is not like that. It can only be derived by painstaking experimentation that first improves our understanding of fundamen-tal stem cell properties. Then by careful and calculated trial-and-error, using the most ingenious techniques imaginable, we might be able to manipulate cells to alter their natural behavior in a beneficial way. This is a daunting challenge. Many of the brightest minds around the world are actively engaged in research, trying to unlock these mysteries of nature and to find applications for the benefit of mankind. But medical and scientific research is slow and difficult. Nobel worthy experiments are rare, but those are sustained by the plethora of unseen and unheralded diligent research activities of thousands of specialists, who provide bits and pieces of the founda-tion and all the supporting structures that allow the spectacular pin-nacles of scientific breakthroughs to emerge.

Stem Cell Medicine will yield results. How big and how far-reach-ing those will be remains to be seen. But all medical eyes are on that research and so are the hopes of many families affected by serious chronic illnesses that seem to have no real solutions but only the prospect of regenerative medicine. Such hopes remain alive and well.

Inventions will come ... but in the meantime, we should take advan-tage of the discoveries already made. SC Nutrition offers a proven practical intervention that anyone concerned about optimizing health and wellness can apply today.

Natural Intervention as Prevention

The prospects of SC Medicine are so dramatic and exciting, especially when heralded in the popular media, that it almost sounds like science fiction. After all, if stem cells can differentiate into almost any cell type, it is possible, in principle at least, to use them to regenerate new 'spare parts' on demand for any part of the body in need. So we are left to imagine stroke victims with restored cranial nerves; paraplegics with new sections of spinal cord; or diabetics with new functioning pancreatic islets; heart attack victims with restored cardiac muscle fibers producing smooth forceful contractibility; or clinically blind victims with new rods and cones in the retina restoring sight. The list goes on and on. No wonder the public is so enthused and engaged, not to mention the manipulation by politicians and other interest groups seeking to advance their individual agendas.

But let us not be misled. We are a long way off from any widespread application of new biotechnology that will afford these kinds of dramatic heroics of regenerative medicine. And SC Nutrition does not even appear on this radar screen. Even the concept of consuming any natural product to produce any such miraculous results is not just grasping at straws, it is totally absurd and utterly ridiculous.

However, what SC Nutrition does not offer in depth and drama, it provides in broad scope and with good sense. This natural intervention is best regarded as a source of prevention. Results have already shown that the prognosis of patients with a wide variety of illnesses (like cardiovascular disease,[1] muscular dystrophy,[2] pulmonary arterial hypertension,[3] arthritis,[4] atherosclerosis,[5] systemic lupus erythematosis,[6] kidney failure[7] and migraines[8]) relate directly to the number of circulating stem cells. In addition, we can now appreciate that many slow degenerative diseases (like Parkinson's, Alzheimer's, diabetes or emphysema) can be associated with the inability of stem cells to adequately regenerate and restore function in the affected tissues. Therefore, the ability of SC Nutrition to enhance the population of circulating stem cells which can traffick to injured or worn-out tissues, does provide at least a novel but natural intervention as a form of primary prevention. This prospect is immediate, convenient and of universal value. Recall our stem cell mantra.

And then, as if nature would reward our cooperation with an additional bonus, there is now evidence that even the prospect of regeneration is not completely out of the picture where SC Nutrition is applied. For example, the regenerative potential of AFA extract has been shown in a mouse model of muscle injury. Mice fed with a specific AFA extract recovered much faster than a control group after an injury to the anterior tibialis muscle[9].

But the bottom line remains. **The number of circulating stem cells does seem to provide a significant marker to establish overall risk to health and the prospect for improving prognosis.** Since SC Nutrition does provide a simple, safe and convenient approach to increasing the number of circulating stem cells, it cannot but help to promote optimal health. Its application could only reflect uncommon wisdom.

Health before Disease

Optimal health must always be the goal. That is valid for everybody, everywhere, everyday. Whatever the circumstance, the objective should always be to minimize illness and disease, to reduce suffering and pain, and to avoid the ultimate death. That is a downward spiral but unfortunately, it is the practical paradigm of medicine. So we search for diagnosis, devise management protocols that apply therapeutics and surgery to reverse the perceived downward trend. That is the disease model. It begins with illness and ends hopefully with recovery. SC Medicine is in search of possible applications of stem cell science and technology to accomplish just that.

Not so with SC Nutrition. Before the appearance of any defined clinical illness, and after the complete recovery from whatever ails the individual, there remains the prospect of optimizing health by enhancing stem cell release and trafficking to tissues that need recovery and restoration. **SC Nutrition is a positive intervention, best understood and appreciated as a protector and preserver of life at its best and health in its most robust state.**

This is a different paradigm. It may or may not serve the best interest of insurance companies, pharmaceutical manufacturers, perhaps some in the medical establishment, and even special interest groups with political agendas. But it definitely does serve the highest and best interests of the individual. To focus on being healthy and remaining so is far better for both the psychology and the physiology of each person. It allows one to be both positive and proactive. Daily support of your natural healing system, enhancing your innate stem cells in their normal restorative and regenerative roles with SC Nutrition, is clearly one of the best personal strategies to remaining healthy. And all of that makes consummate sense *before* any apparent illness strikes. '*An ounce of prevention is worth much more than a pound of cure.*' As such, a truer proverb has never been said.

If and when illness does strike, both the application of medicine *and* nutrition becomes important. The focus may shift from one to the other as the illness progresses from acute to chronic. But in any case, nutrition remains crucial. SC Nutrition can influence recovery and prognosis going forward, as more stem cells are released from the bone marrow, traffick to affected tissues and carry out their normal renewal function.

The take home message in this regard is to favor cell regeneration in a positive way and to support health by promoting and maintaining this optimal tissue renewal, rather than focusing on disease processes. If SC Medicine is regarded as the next best hope for curing disease (when that is the focus, as useful and valid as that may be in the field of medicine), then at the same time and perhaps leading the way in ready application, **SC Nutrition is the best new strategy for optimizing health today.** We need not wait for tomorrow.

Universal Application

When you think of it, at any given time, only a small fraction of the population is acutely ill, or suffering from some debilitating condition that precludes them from getting to work or enjoying their families. Perhaps over ninety percent of the population at any time is waking up prepared for a normal day with regular routines at home, at work or at school. But our passion for SC Medicine is driven by our compassion for loved ones who suffer daily with chronic conditions for which there is little hope of recovery or release. And what is more, we entertain the foreboding prospect that our day will come. If and when our turn comes to endure some unfortunate illness or disease, we would wish for the possibility of new SC Medicine to be available for our potential restoration. That provides some hope and comfort even while SC Medicine is yet to deliver in broad significant ways.

On the contrary, SC Nutrition today attracts little attention and less excitement. The natural renewal system of the body is neglected and taken for granted. In fact, in most cases, there is little or no awareness that **everybody has stem cells; everybody uses stem cells; everybody uses stem cells every day; stem cells work ... and they work every time.**

But widespread awareness becomes necessary for widespread application to be utilized. The message that adult stem cells leave the bone marrow, circulate and migrate into tissues to effect renewal, repair and regeneration needs to be propagated. Plus the availability of safe natural products to enhance this normal renewal process needs to be promoted far and wide.

Whenever it comes to medicine – and here the temptation may be to include SC Nutrition – it would seem that one must always wait to find a basis for therapeutic indication to give a green light to proceed. And the opposite is also true, that one must always be cautious and take time to look for known contra-indications so that one could perceive the red light which demands a stop. That is wisdom in daily medical practice. Only some fools would callously disregard such control signs and rush in where wiser professionals would fear to tread. To do otherwise, is to tempt fate, risk many potential adverse consequences and therefore court a possible disaster waiting to happen.

This is definitely not the case with SC Nutrition. The stem cell mantra we have reiterated underscores that this finds universal application. Everybody is invited to participate. There are hardly any known practical contra-indications in this case. Everyone shares in this novel opportunity to help optimize their health condition by supporting the natural renewal and healing system of the body. You can go beyond the mere absence of illness or disease to enable your body to achieve its optimal state of health by this simple lifestyle choice. If you already suffer in some way or other, you can harness this same renewal system to intensify your struggle to improve and recover. There is nothing to fear.

Food Sources aren't Drugs

Whatever breakthroughs do emerge for SC Medicine, we can be certain of one thing -- pharmaceutical and/or biotechnology companies are almost inevitably destined to capitalize on these innovations and to control accessibility to new therapeutic interventions. That is their legitimate business. Such competitiveness for exclusive patent rights and the desire to capture market share have served the public quite well in the development of major advances in all fields of medicine, and for many years.

Fortunately, however, SC Nutrition is not restricted in any such way. Nutrition is accessible to all. **Anyone can tap into what nature affords to derive whatever benefits are to be gained.** There are limited protective rights and no exclusivity in the normal exploitation of simple, common edible products such as AFA concentrate. Just think of it.

And yet, what is the obvious strength of SC Nutrition may also be its perceived weakness. The public is programmed to anticipate breakthroughs in science and medicine to come about in large sophisticated laboratories filled with great numbers of illustrious scientific researchers in white lab coats. This type of innovation is presented at news conferences with the media spotlight on distinguished pioneers in their field of expertise or else announced in the media by reporters quoting (and often misquoting) from peer-reviewed original articles published in prestigious journals. Then – and only then - the public is duly impressed. Public opinion is manipulated and most patients respond with good compliance when professionals prescribe and dispense whatever new therapeutic product or intervention is being heralded. That's medicine in the modern world.

How could any development in healthcare, derived from any common algae anywhere, anytime, be accepted as a credible breakthrough that can help any ordinary person to experience optimal health or wellness? That is too commonplace for the general public. It appears to lack professional authority and serious scientific credibility. If only it were a new drug, a product of intensive research, produced by a large multinational pharmaceutical company, adver-tised on television with the best of Madison Avenue commercials – then perhaps it would gain ready acceptance everywhere. But it would not change the facts where nature is concerned.

We should always be careful not to confuse hype with substance or image with reality. **The intrinsic properties of nature sometimes overwhelm the best of human efforts and deliver benefits to humankind that at times, no technology can produce.** This has been the contention of alternative/complementary health practition-ers for decades. Just think of all the natural remedies that have had universal appeal, with acclaimed benefits for hundreds of years and more. What of ordinary chicken soup, a warm glass of milk, that one apple-a-day, all the common effective herbal remedies, lemon juice, glucosamine, a shot of brandy ... and the list goes on. Science may only explain what nature will provide even before (and sometimes without) human understanding.

The source of SC Nutrition is no drug but its benefits exceed what many a drug would do. It cooperates with nature, exploiting the natural renewal system of the body with proven advantage to each individual who chooses to indulge.

Biology or Biotechnology

SC Nutrition and SC Medicine can be contrasted in yet another inter-esting way.

Many medical interventions and especially the use of prescription drugs, are aimed at solving some particular biological problem. Usually, a specific drug is designed to target receptor sites on a given cell type, organ or tissue where it produces characteristic pharmaco-logical action that is desired. That approach is eminently reasonable. But almost every drug has unintended consequences, most of which are limited, although some can lead to contraindications that necessarily restrict their use.

One of the principal reasons for the long intensive training of medical doctors is the fact that prescribing drugs with several different points of action and a wide variety of biological responses, requires broad knowledge and practical experience. Of the many drugs that doctors encounter and utilize almost daily, most of them require pages and pages of fine print in the doctor's 'drug bible' (for example, the PDR in the US or the CPS in Canada.) Those references almost universally address issues of indications and contraindications, adverse or side effects, drug interactions, restricted dosages and other special precautions. It is as if one who is distressed will always be in a danger zone, a veritable mine field of biotechnology, trying to locate a place of refuge to find some relief.

Stem Cell Medicine promises to be no different. In the future, we anticipate that stem cells could be harnessed from the same patient (in one form or another) possibly cultured and further manipulated in one or more ways, then reintroduced to the same patient (or to another). Other possibilities certainly exist. Perhaps for example, stem cells could be treated *in* situ in the same patient by some therapeutic intervention or other. This may be local treatment to specific tissues or systemic treatment applied through the circulation. There are stem cell approaches yet to be conceived.

Whatever the biotechnology that exploits the intrinsic properties of stem cells to therapeutic advantage, again we can be sure that the same issues will arise. There will be indications and contraindications, adverse side effects, drug interactions and a host of special precautions. Inevitably, there will be safeguards to limit rejection of any transplanted cells and to minimize any potential development of unwanted tumors, benign or malignant.

SC Nutrition by contrast is essentially biology at work. It is so natural that it invites widespread application. It may not be dramatic intervention at all, but what it lacks in excitement and sensationalism, it makes up in simplicity, convenience and safety. Like normal daily nutrition that is practiced by everybody, everywhere, everyday, it is only biology at work, no more and no less. It remains unencumbered by all the perils and problems that inevitably associate with biotechnology. **In the end, nature knows best, nature does it best and nature provides the best antidotes to satisfy its own needs.**

The goal of SC Nutrition is only to enhance the normal cell renewal process. When more stem cells are released into the bloodstream and they traffick to tissues in need, they require no education or further information. **Circulating stem cells know exactly what their mission is and they tend to perform flawlessly.** They need no precautionary advice to direct or limit their activity. They simply execute consistent with their normal biology.

Diagnostic Medicine, Holistic Nutrition

The practice of modern medicine is developed around a fairly universal paradigm of care. Here's the simple outline. A patient presents to the doctor's office or at the hospital with a *Chief Complaint.* That's the doctor's first focus of question. What is it? How long has it been there? What precipitating factor(s) may have caused it? Etc. That's designed to delineate the *History of the Present Illness.* This is crucial to getting an immediate handle on the problem and good doctors take great care to elicit the pertinent information as accurately and completely as possible. Further questions might provide a quick *Review of Systems.* Then follows a systematic inquiry into the patient's *Past Medical History.* This too is extremely informative. Next is the question of *Family History* to identify increased risks of disease or conditions that may have hereditary factors to consider. Usually this is followed by an enumeration of *Drugs* that the patient is presently taking or has recently taken and of course any known *Allergies* that would be precautionary. Sometimes one would conclude the history taking with an inquiry into *Lifestyle Factors* that may be pertinent such as smoking, sexual habits, domestic living conditions, etc. All this may seem to indicate a long and tedious inquiry but with experience and depending on the circumstances, good doctors conduct a thorough but targeted history in just a few minutes in many situations. At times it could be quite lengthy though, especially with elderly patients, the chronically ill, others with language difficulties, new patients to a practice, etc.

The history then gives rise to a *Physical Examination* which is conducted systematically, again focused but thorough, to identify objective *signs* of illness to complement the subjective symptoms reported by the patient or their attendees. When this is completed, the doctor typically frames a so-called *Differential Diagnosis* which is a list of possible explanations that account for the patient's signs and symptoms. These are generally prioritized.

Armed with all this information, the doctor then selects a series of *laboratory and other Diagnostic Tests* to help to further elucidate and hopefully pin down a *Definitive Diagnosis.* In the meantime a *Management Plan* is devised. When test results are reported, the management plan is revised to reflect the new information and the necessary *therapeutics, treatments, surgeries* or other interventions are executed and followed up. Hopefully, things go well for the patient and another successful case is documented, with plans for future *Follow-up.*

So what's the point here?

The point is very specific. **Medicine is practiced by the pursuit of definitive diagnosis and subsequent treatment of the same.** In the absence of symptoms and signs of illness or disease, there is little basis to specify any definitive diagnosis and therefore little justification for medical intervention.

Not so with nutrition. Long before any symptoms or signs become evident, the body has real needs. There is the constant maintenance of good health, the regular repair of damaged and worn out tissues and organs, and the constant growth and development appropriate for every age and stage of life. For all these consistent and potential activities, **nutrition is not just important or even vital, it is indispensable**. Regular daily adequate intake of nutrients is a *sine qua non*.

SC Nutrition falls into that same category. The normal and natural renewal system of the body is consistently at work in support of *all* the tissues of the body and in the promotion of optimal health and wellness. The opportunity to enhance this intrinsic and essential repair system, naturally empowers any individual to take responsibility and to cultivate this convenient lifestyle habit to much advantage, wherever and whenever possible.

Not for Professionals Only

SC Nutrition is therefore not to be dispensed from behind the pharmacy counter or to be picked up at the family doctor's office. There is no such restriction or limitation. On the contrary, it could be made available and accessible to all, without discrimination with respect to medical history or to clinical condition.

Here is an opportunity for the ordinary person to utilize a rather ordinary natural product, derived from ordinary sources such as the wild-harvested, certified organic, microalgae, *Aphanizomenon flos-aquae* (AFA), to influence the ordinary health renewal system of the human body. But that ordinary lifestyle habit could lead to extraordinary possibilities and potential consequences. Since the number of circulating stem cells in the body is a marker or indicator of health risk and a contributing factor to progress and prognosis in the face of different types of illness, the ability to increase that number by dietary supplementation is a novel health promotion tool that cannot be disregarded lightly.

But how is the world to know of the wellness transforming possibilities of SC Nutrition?

It's very unlikely to come from the medical establishment. Doctors by and large, are trained to think and act in a certain way. They see the ravages of disease almost daily and cannot but see the world of humanity through that lens. They think of all that could happen to any patient and therefore carry so much responsibility. By training and disposition, they are always careful to consider the worst-case scenario, lest they neglect or overlook a serious clinical threat or condition. After all, patients are just that - patients. They are people with symptoms, complaints, illnesses, diseases ... that all need to be treated or managed. And there is enough of that to keep any doctor busy ... 'stressed by the tyranny of the urgent.' Those individuals who have no pressing complaints may need a psychologist or a counselor. They may need a social worker or ... a nutritionist. But they hardly merit a busy doctor. The Greatest Teacher and Physician of all made the wise observation that **'they that are whole need not a physician, but they that are sick.'** True. No wonder the doctor tends to triage those that appear 'healthy' to the bottom of the list for urgent or thorough attention. And unfortunately, that's where all the lifestyle issues get dumped. That's the time for education and counseling regarding the factors that influence good health and promote wellness. It's not the time for medical attention.

However, there is a major contradiction in all that. Studies have shown that when all the factors that impact the risk of disease, the quality of life and even the length of life are considered, the relative importance of these factors becomes inverted. Here are the best quantitative estimates:

Table 3: Relative factors that influence disease risk and quality of life

Lifestyle	50%
Environment	20%
Genetics	10%
Medical Care	10%

There's another perspective that makes the same point, perhaps more emphatically. Researchers at Harvard School of Public Health, with collaboration from the Universities of Toronto and Washington, also did a comprehensive study to look at how diet, lifestyle and metabolic risk factors for chronic disease contribute to mortality in America[10]. Table 4 summarizes their findings:

Table 4: Annual US Deaths attributed to individual Risk Factors

Smoking	467,000	High dietary salt	103,000
High Blood Pressure	395,000	Low omega-3 FA (diet)	84,000
Overweight/Obesity	216,000	High trans FA (diet)	82,000
Sedentary Lifestyle	191,000	Alcohol abuse	64,000
High blood sugar	190,000	Low fruits & vegetables	58,000
High LDL Cholesterol	113,000	Low PUFA (diet)	15,000

What that adds up to in effect is that over one million premature deaths occur In the United States each year, all caused by modifiable risk factors. Those figures all speak for themselves. We will address the lifestyle issues as they pertain to stem cells in the next chapter but the pattern is clear. The role of medical care is grossly exaggerated when optimal health is either the subject at hand or the goal in view.

The question remains, 'How will the information about SC Nutrition get out into the marketplace best, before people become patients?' How does one convey a message that seems too good to be true? The answer is simple: 'by word-of-mouth'. Surely, professionals can talk to other professionals. Researchers and scientists will share the latest developments with each other, as more evidence is forthcoming. Research publications in the medical and scientific literature will continue to point to the validity and value of the natural healing system of the body, implicating endogenous adult stem cells in a variety of ways.

However, make no mistake about it. The most efficient and effective way to disseminate and apply the information about SC Nutrition is through the ordinary lay person passing on the information to all those within their social sphere of contact and influence. It is an open opportunity for all to participate, using every available means, including social media and the internet. Recall that stem cell mantra one more time. It's all about everybody, everywhere, everyday, using ordinary natural products like those derived from proven algae concentrates of AFA, to enhance stem cell mobilization and trafficking to benefit tissues in need, with anticipated benefits to health. This is not for professionals only. It's for everyone concerned with optimum health and wellness. The risk-benefit analysis favors widespread application and that invites constant person-to-person communication. There's nothing to lose … and a lot to gain!

While sharing the opportunity and benefits of SC Nutrition, there is even more to gain in elaborating the healthful value of a **Stem Cell Lifestyle** in general. That's the subject of the next chapter.

CHAPTER 11

A Stem Cell Lifestyle

In the field of medicine, we learn that many different illnesses and diseases of the body result from or are influenced by a variety of factors acting individually or in concert. As such, they are described as multi-factorial conditions. Take for example, the number one killer in North America, cardiovascular disease (CVD). The known risk factors for this prevalent condition include a positive family history, hypertension, diabetes, hypercholesterolemia, cigarette smoking, stress and a sedentary lifestyle.

Interestingly enough, these same risk factors tend to affect the number of circulating stem cells. In this regard it is now known that the bone marrow-derived endothelial progenitor cells (EPCs) relate to the pathogenesis of atherosclerosis and the progression of CVD. In a study of 135 consecutive hospitalized patients with CVD and 25 healthy subjects, the number of EPCs was less in the patients than in the healthy subjects[1]. Furthermore, that number significantly correlated with the number of risk factors. It was lower in patients with hypertension and diabetes mellitus, and in smokers compared to non smokers among the healthy subjects, but surprisingly not among the patients.

In a quantitative sense, some of those factors are more important than others and the combined risk when more than one is present, tends to be multiplicative rather than additive. From the patient's viewpoint, what is more significant is that personal lifestyle choices can impact most of these risks. Thus, a person can do much to reduce their risk of cardiovascular disease if they are compliant in managing any essential hypertension and achieving good blood sugar and cholesterol control (by at least cooperating with good medical advice). They can do much more also by avoiding smoking, keeping a handle on their weight, learning to manage inordinate stress and getting moderate exercise on a regular basis.

In a nutshell, any individual would do well to adopt such a lifestyle consistent with minimizing the known risk factors for cardiovascular disease. That is why every patient leaving the hospital after a heart attack or stroke is given specific instructions about these very lifestyle issues. And by the way, the doctor is never as eager to give such lifestyle advice and encouragement, and the patients are never as willing to hear and as anxious to comply with the same, as they are after surviving a serious and scary event. These patients are keen to make lifestyle changes, but obviously that is the second best. Those same healthy lifestyle choices would make far better sense and be far more productive and *healthful* if they were adopted before there was even any evidence of cardiovascular disease.

The essential principles of a 'wellness lifestyle' promise to transform the promotion of optimal health and reduce the incidence of illness and disease. In that regard, patients must take personal responsibility for their health; focus on prevention of illness rather than wait for diagnosis and treatment; employ natural alternatives wherever necessary and effective, and finally, seek to experience integrated health as a 'whole person'.

The case has been made that Stem Cell (SC) Nutrition provides the latest opportunity to transform the 'wellness phenomenon' by focusing on enhancing the body's natural healing and renewal system. That is through increasing the release of stem cells from the bone marrow and their ability to get their job done.

However, that useful intervention through convenient dietary supplementation is ineffective in a vacuum. There are other lifestyle choices that the individual must make to further effect the desired 'optimal wellness' outcome. We can therefore define and describe a so called 'Stem Cell Lifestyle' that focuses on supporting the normal role and functions of stem cells in the body on a daily basis. That goes beyond nutrition and over and above SC Nutrition. **Essentially, the application of SC Nutrition is certainly a wise and welcome lifestyle habit.** It should neither be considered as a conditional alternative to anything else, nor as a complete answer to everything else. It cannot serve as penance to erase all the unhealthy mistakes of the past, nor should it be expected to be a panacea for all the negative consequences of those mistakes to be realized in the future. SC Nutrition could indeed be a major component of any healthful lifestyle, but it would still be only one of the various contributors. There are several others that must be engaged in concert.

Therefore, it is important to examine the so called 'Stem Cell Lifestyle' and to weigh in on the role of other lifestyle choices that can impact the performance of stem cells in the body. The goal is to promote a total wellness lifestyle as a package. After all, that has always been the proper perspective on health. It is never piecemeal or particular in its focus. Rather, the emphasis has always been on the whole person.

Health has always been and always will be a synergistic phenomenon. Since there are component links in the chain that undergirds and protects this invaluable blessing in life, then the adage still remains true that 'no chain is stronger than its weakest link'. **We can never compensate for one unhealthy lifestyle habit by exploiting all the benefits to be derived in some other area.** Nature does reward only integrity and consistency in the lifestyle arena and therefore summons us to responsible behavior, 24/7. That would define the Stem Cell Lifestyle.

So, what would such a Stem Cell Lifestyle actually look like? Surprisingly, (or not really, when all things are considered) some of the same healthy lifestyle choices that are well known to be beneficial and in effect, preventive of illness and disease, turn out to be just as healthful and important with respect to their impact on stem cell behavior.

The opposite of this is also true. Factors such as daily exposure to cigarette smoke and other environmental toxins, physical and mental stress, poor diet and the so-called 'aging process', may all cause a decline in the body's ability to renew itself. Such negative influences could cause a reduction in the release and activity of adult stem cells. This then leads to a decline in the natural ability of the body to maintain optimum health. Therefore, all these become most relevant to any consideration of a Stem Cell Lifestyle.

We choose to begin with the negative in this case, for there is quite an obvious correlation. And almost certainly, the first negative lifestyle indiscretion that probably comes to mind is the habit of smoking. So that's the obvious place to begin.

NO SMOKING

This one is really a no brainer. Just recall the four healthful wellness principles that we discussed in the last chapter and then consider the real implications of cigarette smoking. As a lifestyle habit, it is certainly a derogation of *personal responsibility*. Choosing to smoke may still be exercising a personal right, but it remains an unhealthy choice. It is definitely the opposite of health promotion or sickness/disease *prevention*. On the contrary, it is more a prime causation of major illnesses including the very big ones like cardiovascular disease, lung and throat cancer and COPD (chronic obstructive pulmonary disease). It is an unnatural alternative – the unnecessary inhalation of over 200 toxic chemicals, all foreign to the normal human body. That is absurd, when you think of it. Finally, rather than *supporting the whole person*, it exerts its negative influence on all aspects of human experience. It contaminates the body, subverts and controls the mind, derails the spirit and becomes a social blight that strains relationships and drains the pocketbook. Therefore, on all four counts, smoking gets a failing grade and is consequently repugnant to any wellness lifestyle.

Fortunately, although smoking still remains a fairly widespread habit (in certain communities), the practice has been much in decline - thanks to the concerted efforts of ordinary individuals, many organizations and the US Surgeon General. Add to that, government regulations restricting public advertising and the prevalence of unhealthy consequences that have become an increasing deterrent. Then consider the risk and cost of medical insurability and the outcry against second hand smoke that has made the habit mostly distasteful and unsociable. For all these and other reasons, smoking has essentially become *anathema*.

But there are still pockets of resistance in even the best of communities in North America as well as some die-hard cultural forces that continue to perpetuate too high a prevalence of this unhealthy practice. Some stakeholders and special interest groups defend their freedom to choose and therefore lobby and fight to defend their turf. But that is becoming more of a lost cause and the battle is no longer justifiable on any grounds. When one considers the BIG picture, that's really how it ought to be.

By the way, smoking cannabis (marijuana) is no better. The idea of any medical marijuana use may have its place in palliative care in some circumstances, but the ongoing or casual use of this drug can hardly be justified for any reason as a healthful lifestyle habit. At best, it does little for the integration of personal physiological performance and at worst, it increases the risk for abuse of other substances that are unambiguously destructive to health optimization or any wellness objective. To put it bluntly, smoking marijuana - just like smoking cigarettes- has no place in a Stem Cell Lifestyle now, or any time in the future for that matter.

So what is the stem cell connection to smoking?

First, we must appreciate that the normal lung has a number of repair cells, called fibroblasts that effectively undergo continuous proliferation to repair the ongoing natural process of degeneration. These tissue stem cells will typically divide 30-50 times before the multiplication process is arrested by some kind of cellular exhaustion. This arrest is referred to as 'replicative senescence'. In mathematical terms, one such stem cell undergoing a cycle of 30 divisions would generate over 6,000,000,000 (billion) new cells. That represents an amazing regenerative capacity for stem cells in the lung.

Repair processes appear to be quite active in the normal lung. The magnitude of this tissue repair is suggested by the observation that as much as 5% of the lung collagen, for example, can turn over in the adult animal on a daily basis[2]. Maintenance of normal tissue structure (so important for lung function, especially in the tiny alveolar spaces) requires that the amount of newly synthesized collagen balances the amount of degraded collagen. That is consistent with active repair of damaged tissue in the normal lung.

However, in the case of chronic smokers, the damage to lung tissue is accelerated and more widespread. Therefore the pulmonary effects naturally include increased risks for cancer and COPD, both of which can have serious, if not fatal consequences. The pathogenesis of lung cancer has been directly linked to toxic carcinogens like nicotine. That case is now closed and the repercussions are far-reaching, but personal application is what really matters now. At the same time, and unfortunately, COPD does not get the attention it deserves. It is the fourth leading cause of death in North America and cigarette smoking is perhaps the major culprit.

Classically, emphysema (a type of COPD that is definitely linked to smoking) is believed to develop when mediators of tissue injury exceed the protective mechanisms within the lung. Such tissue destruction then represents an imbalance between tissue injury and repair. Cigarette smoke can be toxic to cells within the lung and can impede the repair functions of fibroblasts (as well as epithelial and mesenchymal cells) through both direct and indirect pathways. Of note, cigarette smoke extracts (CSEs) were shown to reduce the ability of stem cells to migrate to lung tissue and then to proliferate and differentiate into (pulmonary) lung cells[3].

The lung fibroblasts in patients with COPD show a reduced growth rate compared to the lungs of non COPD patients. A single exposure to CSE inhibits the normal fibroblast proliferation even further. But multiple exposures to CSE move these cells into an irreversible state of premature cellular senescence. This has a profound effect on the ability of these stem cells to accomplish their work of regeneration and repair in the compromised lung[4].

Canadian researchers at Mount Sinai Hospital in Toronto have demonstrated that volatile components of cigarette smoke inhibit the normal repair responses of epithelial cells present in the airways of smokers[5]. In another recent study out of Switzerland, researchers found that cigarette smoke does inhibit lung fibroblast proliferation by mechanisms suggestive of changes in translation of mRNA (messenger RNA)[6].

When stem cells were grown in culture, exposure to 5% fresh CSEs reduced growth by a half and similar exposure to 10% CSEs stopped this proliferation completely. However (and most encouraging of all), the effect was reversible after discontinuing the exposure to CSEs, although not completely so. Similar results related to these scenarios were obtained with respect to the migration ability of lung stem cells[7].

A further interesting observation relates to the deleterious effects of second hand smoke. When mouse embryonic stem cells (ESCs) were exposed alternatively to actual CSEs and to an extract of secondary smoke, the effect of the latter was greater in the inhibition of growth, differentiation and survival of the mouse ESCs[8].

So much for the lungs. Cigarette smoking has other serious damaging health consequences. As mentioned earlier, it is a leading risk factor for cardiovascular disease (North America's #1 killer). In fact, it accounts for almost 50% of coronary events. But here's the good news - the risk of heart attack or stroke decreases by a similar 50% within the first two years after smoking cessation[9].

Chronic smokers have endothelial dysfunction[10]. The inner linings of important blood vessels are prone to lose their integrity and innate reactivity. This endothelial reactivity clearly predicts future cardiac events,[11] but even in chronic smokers, smoking cessation helps to restore endothelial function and reduces future C-V risk[12].

Both experimental and clinical studies showed that endothelial progenitor cells (EPCs) are mobilized from bone marrow in response to tissue ischemia and vascular injury[13]. These mobilized EPCs therefore contribute to not only the birth of new microvasculature but also to endothelial repair of larger blood vessels[14]. A recent study reported that cigarette smoking is associated with fewer circulating stem cells (EPC's) and their impairment to differentiate into functional tissue[15a].

Research out of Japan has demonstrated that the number of circulating EPCs and other progenitor cells (PCs) was reduced in chronic smokers. However, smoking cessation led to a rapid restoration of PC/EPC levels. The recovery was greater in light smokers than in heavy smokers. The implications here of course, are obvious[15b].

When it comes to stem cells and cancer, the harmful effects of smoking and that disease may have secondary implications. Studies examining the impact of smoking in cancer survivor outcomes, have focused on tobacco- related cancers, typically those of the lung, head and neck. Clear associations have been found between smoking and negative outcomes:[16]

i)   reduced efficacy of treatments (chemo- and radio-therapy, surgery)
ii) delayed surgical healing
iii) creation and/or exacerbation of common attendant illnesses
iv) increased risk of secondary cancers and cancer recurrence, and
v)   decreased chances of survival

Treatment of some cancers not directly associated with smoking, such as leukemia, often involves hematopoietic stem cell transplantation. Smoking appears to adversely affect both hospitalization and overall survival in these cases[17]. There is increased risk of respiratory failure mediated in part by abnormal lung function before transplantation and likely through other mechanisms.

Smoking has yet other negative influences on stem cells. In bone healing, for example, there is usually a two-step process: stem cells become cartilage and then that cartilage matures into bone. The same research group at Mount Sinai Hospital in Toronto (referred to earlier) showed just over a decade ago that cigarette smoke inhibits osteogenic differentiation and proliferation of human osteo-progenitor (bone stem) cells. In simple terms, stem cells from the bone marrow were much less capable of forming new bone[18].

In another study, researchers at the University of Rochester identified nicotine as the culprit responsible for delaying bone growth by influencing gene expression in the two-step process alluded to prior. Further study identified a second smoke ingredient, the poly-aromatic hydrocarbon benzo (a) pyrene (BaP) as another villain slowing bone healing, though by a different mode of action[19].

There is no doubt that if Stem Cell Nutrition has appeal to those who would value optimal wellness as an extremely high priority, then **cigarette smoking would find no place whatsoever in a Stem Cell Lifestyle.** It is preventable behavior with very high disease risk, and with significant attendant morbidity. In today's world, the social stigma now associated with the habit and the effective technology and medical management designed to facilitate quitting, all offer hope to anyone who chooses to adopt a new value system and an appropriate healthful way of life.

We turn next to another major contributor to quality of life and health, namely, the management of inordinate stress.

MANAGED STRESS

Stress is itself a blessing and yet a curse. It is *the physiological adaptation syndrome designed by nature to allow human beings especially to cope with threats and challenges that demand quick and alert, energetic and efficient response for maximum personal advantage.* That's this author's definition but it correlates with Dr Hans Selye's original ideas when he first formulated the basics of this field.

Stress should not be measured by excitement, misfortune, productivity or responsibility. These are contributing factors that only set the stage for the individual actor to perform. It is the response to all of the above and more, that quantifies the *amount* of stress and qualifies the *nature* of the stress experienced. Therefore the relevant issue and the appropriate phrase we choose to use with respect to health and wellness is the **'management of inordinate stress'**. There are two key words to underline here. 'Inordinate' implies that the stress is either unnecessary, exaggerated, misplaced or unusually burdensome. It often results from anxiety (conflict of values or objectives), overwork (from attempting too much, too fast or expecting perfection), or selfish preoccupation (from failure to share, serve or surrender). The second word is 'management'. That implies careful, deliberate, structured and controlled response that avoids over reacting, worrying or capitulating. It is learning to set limits, to say 'no', to define personal boundaries, to delegate, to pace oneself, to breathe, to relax and to sleep. All that and more is involved in managing stress.

Having said all that, we must still acknowledge that chronic stress (which is poorly managed inordinate stress) is a personal lifestyle habit or disposition adopted by far too many people. That is not good. Chronic stress over-stimulates the adrenal glands, pumping high levels of adrenalin into the bloodstream and overdriving the autonomic nervous system. This all leads to a variety of ill effects such as hypertension, heart disease, ulcers, weight changes, depressed immunity, insomnia, skin disorders, hair loss unintentional tremors, migraine headaches, and digestive tract disorders.

So what does all that mean for stem cells? In a word, poorly managed inordinate stress can suppress the ability of stem cells to perform their normal continuous function of natural healing and repair in the body.

Some Japanese scientists studied neural stem cell kinetics in rats that were exposed to chronic stress conditions[20]. They found that stress reduced the ability of stem cells in the brain to proliferate. They were able to demonstrate that this effect was directly related to elevated stress hormone (adrenalin, noradrenalin) levels because the effect could be eliminated by surgically removing the animals' adrenal glands. That's the downside. In contrast to that negative effect, when brain stem cells were grown *in vitro*, the addition of the 'happy neurotransmitter' serotonin increased their survival. This all suggests that at least one mechanism by which chronic stress can affect health might be by reducing the ability of stem cells to proliferate and do what they do best – normal healing and repair of tissues.

In an earlier study, other Japanese researchers showed that in humans, the stress of surgery inhibited the growth of fibroblasts (stem cells in the skin) through the elevation of stress hormone (catecholamines and cortisol) levels in the blood stream[21]. This elevation of stress hormones is typical for post-op patients who must endure the burdens of anesthesia, surgical incision and manipulation and physical invasion (as purposeful as it all might be). In this study, serum was collected from patients a few days after surgery. When fibroblasts were exposed to this post-op serum, their proliferation was suppressed. This could be perhaps typical of a more general phenomenon whereby the effect of stress – surgical or otherwise – is to depress the natural healing system of the body. The normal physiological function of stem cells may be negatively impacted by chronic stress through some mechanism(s) that impede proliferation and differentiation in different tissues.

Therefore in pursuit of optimal wellness, **the Stem Cell Lifestyle demands deliberate management of inordinate stress**. It does not imply the avoidance of challenge or responsibility, personal initiative or productive work. It does require careful focus on the things that really matter and that is, 'avoiding the tyranny of the urgent' while embracing 'the stewardship of what's really important'.

POSITIVE MENTAL ATTITUDE

Managing stress is closely associated with one's overall mental attitude. Before we engage in any activity, our daily approach to life with all its inherent vicissitudes is a critical determinant in both the quality of life itself and the attainment of optimal wellness. Positive people tend to enjoy not only the benefit of a winsome personality, but they do themselves a big favor by up-regulating their immune system, calming or stabilizing their nervous system and even slowing down their natural process of aging.

This general phenomenon that is witnessed everywhere and every day, has given rise to a whole new field of inquiry that has now become an infant science with a long descriptive name: Psychoneuroimmunology. Studies are now appearing in scientific literature that link attitudes and states of mind, plus the experience and level of emotions, with the physical performance of the central nervous system as well as the immune system.

The celebrated author Norman Cousins perhaps opened the door to this new field with his classic 1979 book, *"Anatomy of an Illness - as Perceived by the Patient"*. In the book he described for the benefit of all, his reflections on healing and regeneration. He illustrated the concept at the heart of the holistic approach to health. He argued that the human mind is capable of promoting the body's potential for healing itself even when faced with a seemingly hopeless medical predicament. He recounted his personal experiences of working in close collaboration with his doctor to overcome a crippling and supposedly irreversible disease. He was a distinguished journalist and peace activist who outlined the life-saving and ultimately life-prolonging benefit to be gained by taking responsibility for one's own well being. Here's how he put it himself, *"I have learned never to underestimate the capacity of the human mind and body to regenerate – even when the prospects seem most wretched"*. He championed the power of 'laughter as the best medicine'. Again he wrote from his own experience, *"I made the joyous discovery that ten minutes of genuine belly laughter had an anesthetic effect and would give me at least two hours of pain free sleep".*

Cousins suffered a massive heart attack in 1980 and wrote a second masterpiece *"The Healing Heart"* in which he details the events leading up to the attack, the importance of coping with panic, the treatment process, his intensive rehabilitation program and his ultimate recovery. What a testimony to the holistic and complementary approach to illness and health. After his experiences as an adjunct faculty member at the UCLA School of Medicine, Professor Cousins later published *"Headfirst – The Biology of Hope and the Healing Power of the Human Spirit"* (1990). He showed how an optimistic outlook and a strong relationship with one's doctor can make illness less painful and increase one's chances of survival. This is good medicine for all. Despite his painful crippling arthritis and long history of heart disease, he managed to live to age 75.

Positive mental attitude is totally consistent with the Stem Cell Lifestyle. We know that stem cells belong to the same broad class as immune cells. They both are reactive to stimulating molecules (chemokines) that cause them to proliferate and differentiate on demand. We also know that many immune cells have various receptors for neurotransmitters (NTs) like dopamine, noradrenalin and serotonin on their membrane surface[22]. Therefore one would anticipate that such immune cells would respond to emotional states that trigger NT release. Consider the effect of stress, for example, which often involves emotional reaction. And stress is known to definitely suppress immune function [23].

Furthermore, some of the smaller blood vessels (arterioles and capillaries) are known to have nerve terminals that release NTs which attract immune cells or modulate their activity[24]. These nerve terminals prove to be essential for different immune reactions which can be affected if and when certain NTs are blocked[25]. This provides a physical link between the nervous system (brain activity) and the cells of the immune system. One would therefore again anticipate a similar association between the 'emotions of the brain' and stem cells.

A strong hint of this can be derived from at least one study using the famous 'knockout mice'. Researchers showed that the nervous system could somehow regulate the mobilization of stem cells from the bone marrow. In one case they used drugs to block the release of noradrenalin and in the other they genetically removed the ability to maintain the normal neurotransmission of noradrenalin. They found that in either case, stem cell release from the bone marrow was inhibited even when stimulated by G-CSF. On the contrary, stem cell release was enhanced by administering NTs that mimic noradrenalin[26]. (Could the effect here be in contrast to the stress response because the mechanisms relate to NTs as opposed to hormones in the latter case? One would think so.)

These results are interesting but preliminary. More research is needed in this new field. But it is tempting to speculate that positive mental attitude and creative visualization techniques could, in principle, lead to activation of nerve terminals in specific areas of the body that might then support migration of stem cells toward particular tissues in need. Activation of small blood vessels and local microvasculature by some similar means might further assist in targeting stem cell renewal and repair in some areas of concentration. That's a futuristic prospect.

MODERATE EXERCISE

The benefits of exercise are more talked about and observed by others than they are actually enjoyed by the population at large – especially in affluent societies. Sports and physical exercise have become primarily entertainment and as such, few tend to participate on the field of action, while many are content to sit and watch from the spectator stands, or at home on the sofa in front of the television. In any case, millions are missing out.

Frequent and regular physical exercise boosts the immune system and helps protect against cardiovascular disease, Type II diabetes and obesity - the newest modern epidemic. Exercise also improves mental health, builds self-esteem and helps fight depression. Nature provides much encouragement of this healthy lifestyle habit by rewarding active participants with the sensual thrill of 'endogenous morphine' – increasing release of natural endorphins and a more recently identified neurotransmitter, anandamide. These give rise to the exercise-induced euphoria that encourages exercise enthusiasts even further. It can even become addictive. And in this case, that's an addiction that is positive!

Effects of exercise on stem cells seem to be reserved for the really committed fitness 'fanatics'. Those who engage in light or moderate activity seem to have been left out by nature from this extra special recognition and reward. But marathoners, in particular, are selected for this limited prize. Sports physiologists have found that the number of circulating stem cells in the blood of marathon runners is increased by a factor of four (4) after completing a run[27]. They also found increases in levels of G-CSF and interleukin -6, both of which are known cytokines (chemicals) involved in stem cell release from the bone marrow. The stimulating effect remained for a full day, but the stem cell levels returned to their typical baseline numbers by the next day. Similar tests on rowers engaged in very intense rowing exercises showed a different set of results[28]. The level of circulating stem cells remained unchanged, whereas blood cytokines were found to increase.

Clearly, exercise is not all beneficial to the body. There is a price to pay ('*no pain, no gain*'). In the case of extreme exercise like running a marathon, it is obvious that tissues get injured and abused[29]. This triggers release of cytokines, especially G-CSF, that enhance the release of stem cells from the bone marrow that then go on a recovery mission. They traffick to injured tissues and set about repairing and renewing muscles, tendons and ligaments that got strained, damaged or worse during the exercise.

Could it be that all exercise and trauma to the body promotes stem cell release? In the case of marathoners, we might be looking at a difference in *degree* rather than in kind. Maybe the effects are relatively smaller in moderate exercise, or even as seen in the case of intense rowing. But the possibility remains that whenever exercise triggers some level of tissue damage, the natural repair and renewal system of the body (that necessitates stem cell release and trafficking) does become activated to one degree or another. In that case, the normal exercise-induced release of stem cells might be one of the mechanisms of action by which exercise promotes health outcomes. Regardless, **the benefits of moderate exercise are too many and too good to be missed as part of a normal Stem Cell Lifestyle.** (Moderate exercise may be assumed to be that which elevates resting heart rate by about 50%, for periods of 20 – 30 minutes, two or three times per week). Moderate exercise has one further benefit of note – it helps to regulate sleep.

ADEQUATE SLEEP

No one doubts the healthful value of good sleep. It is critical to life itself and a cornerstone of overall wellness. Shakespeare wrote centuries ago in *Macbeth:*

> *"Sleep that knits up the raveled sleeve of troubled care,*
> *Balm of hurt minds, sore labor's bath".*

He got that right, like he did so much else.

Indeed, sleep is an antidote for much that ails and strains the human condition. It is restorative and re-creative, refreshing the soul and renewing mind and body. Yet in our overworked, high-strung, fast paced, anxious and worrisome society, sleep disorders are not uncommon. Just reflect on the use and abuse of hypnotics (sleeping pills), anxiolytics, (antianxiety drugs), and tranquilizers. In the affluence of North American society, we have become a restless, sleep-deprived people. We are over-stimulated by stress and overburdened by worry and care.

The Stem Cell Lifestyle that pursues optimal wellness demands that we get adequate sleep. The word 'adequate' is key, for it depends on each individual's circumstances and need. Perhaps the best measure of adequacy is the experience of awaking from sleep. Adequate sleep results in a feeling of tranquility and alertness on awaking. There is no drowsiness, fatigue or somnolence throughout the day (except for those who cat-nap for short intervals at different times, by choice and not of necessity). Finally, adequate sleep results in a gentle but speedy falling off to sleep at night to crown a good day's work.

For a long time, it seemed reasonable to assume that adequate sleep would affect stem cells in a positive way. Patients who sleep better, should fare better. They should recover faster and just have better outcomes following almost every illness or medical condition. Is there any evidence to support these ideas? In one study, some patients who received bone marrow transplants were observed to recover much faster when they experienced good sleep following the procedure[30]. That led researchers to propose that deep sleep might promote stem cell proliferation and recovery through the production of growth hormone (increased during sleep) and possibly other mechanisms. Deep sleep refers to classic rapid-eye-movement (REM) sleep, the period during which growth hormone production is at its peak. In animal models, growth hormone promotes the proliferation of bone marrow stem cells, which is all consistent with the patient observations.

A second hormone produced particularly during sleep is melatonin. This hormone is produced by the pineal gland, a small endocrine gland located in the center of the brain, but outside the blood-brain barrier. It forms part of the system regulating the sleep-wake cycle because it chemically influences drowsiness and lowers body temperature. However, that cycle is controlled by other CNS (central nervous system) nuclei. Melatonin is more than a hormone. It is also a powerful free radical scavenger and a broad spectrum antioxidant that does not undergo redox cycling.

Melatonin is known to support immune function and also stimulate the secretion of G-CSF. You will recall that G-CSF is well known to trigger stem cell release from the bone marrow. Melatonin has been shown to support the proliferation of bone marrow stem cells[31]. Although no studies have reported the effect of sleep on stem cell mobilization, it is quite reasonable to conclude that sleep (and probably rest, in general) does lead to higher melatonin levels. This produces higher G-CSF in circulation which stimulates stem cell mobilization. That finally enhances tissue renewal and repair when illness or injury is present.

Adequate sleep therefore holds its rightful place and deserves proper emphasis in any consideration of a Stem Cell Lifestyle that purports to promote optimal wellness.

That leaves us with the *pièce de résistance* of the Stem Cell Lifestyle -Complete and Balanced Nutrition including supplementation.

COMPLETE AND BALANCED NUTRITION

We already made the case for complete and balanced nutrition, including supplementation, back in Chapter 4. In the discussion of a Stem Cell Lifestyle, there is only the necessity to consider how nutrition can impact stem cells directly. Throughout the book we have referred to Stem Cell Nutrition to imply any dietary means to enhance stem cell mobilization.

That of course begins with supplementation by stem cell enhancers, of which a synergistic combination of a specific AFA concentrate and a specific fucoidan concentrate leads the way. It has been demonstrated that ingestion of moderate amounts (1 to 1.5gm) of such a formulation provides a ready response enhancing the release of some 20-30% more stem cells (a few million) into the peripheral circulation. As we saw in Chapter 6, the mild but significant effect persists typically for several hours.

Stem Cell Nutrition does not end there. We saw back in Chapter 2 and again in Chapter 6, that both the processes of inflammation and oxidative stress can impede the proper function of stem cells. It is also known that there are many natural edible products that contain useful ingredients with pronounced anti-inflammatory and antioxidant properties. Therefore, there is certainly a role for nutrition in helping to reduce the negative influences resulting from ordinary inflammation and oxidative stress.

Medical students learn in first year pathology that inflammation may be defined as '*the body's natural response to injury*'. During that response, local tissues secrete cytokines as messengers to get help[32]. Among them, SDF-1 is the most important to stem cells. Those 'rescue and repair' cells are attracted to SDF-1 like a magnet. That's fine. But here's the dilemma. Low- grade chronic inflammation leads to constant release of cytokines from different parts of the body. This leads to low levels of SDF-1 spread diffusedly across many different tissues. As a result, stem cells would tend to be recruited constantly into these areas of persistent low-grade inflammation. Other cytokines from these areas can diffuse through the circulation to further trigger more inflammation in other areas. The net effect is that chronic inflammation leads to its systemic dissemination. This causes SDF-1 to also diffuse in the circulation, drawing stem cells away from the microvasculature where it can migrate out into tissues with more acute need. Thus, chronic inflammation tends to reduce both the *quantity* of stem cells available for local, acute renewal and repair, and the *efficiency* of those same stem cells to migrate effectively to points of more urgent need.

That being the case, compounds that help maintain healthy inflammation levels as part of SC Nutrition, provide an important and effective means to increase availability of stem cells for healing and repair. They also improve their migration ability where it counts. Such natural compounds might include phycocyanin, devil's claw, ginger, curcumin, cat's claw or bromelain. With their healthy inflammation properties, they can assist stem cell trafficking by reducing general systemic inflammation. Minor sites become no longer attractive and distracting to stem cells on their mission. Instead, those cells are more discriminating. They recognize the sites in need (where cytokines continue to be secreted), migrate more efficiently into those tissues and finally get the job done.

Oxidative stress presents a similar challenge. Stem cells migrate primarily from post- capillary venules – the tiny vessels between the fine capillaries and the tiniest veins. As you might recall from Chapter 6, these can become blocked by the formation of a fibrin mesh (agglomerate) in the early stages of the coagulation cascade that leads to formation of blood clots. Fibrin is a monomer formed from a larger (dimeric) precursor protein called fibrinogen, under the control of an enzyme protein called thrombrin. Further details aside, fibrinogen is highly susceptible to oxidative modification (about 20 times more so than other plasma proteins like albumen, immunoglobulins or transferrin).

Thus, when the body experiences oxidative stress for whatever reason, fibrinogen is converted more readily to fibrin and those monomers tend to agglomerate and form mesh, not necessarily mature clots. The mesh is adequate to block the microvasculature and impede stem cell migration. Fibrinolytic enzymes like nattokinase and serrapeptase reverse this process and therefore would support the function of stem cells[33].

However, nutrition can help to mitigate this potential problem. Antioxidants in the diet can reduce oxidative stress in the blood and in this way at least, will favor and support stem cell function. But they will do even more. For example, antioxidants extracted from berries and other natural products have been demonstrated to promote the proliferation of human stem cells. Likewise, researchers found that a blend of blueberry, green tea, catechin, carnosine and vitamin D increased the proliferation of bone marrow stem cells by 70% *in vitro*[34]. At least, these results are consistent and in the right direction, and *in vivo* studies would be the logical next step. There is good reason to believe that dietary antioxidants will have one more reason for health recognition because they support the function of stem cells in their normal function of tissue renewal. That's just another indication of the real value of SC Nutrition as part of a SC Lifestyle that aims to produce optimal wellness – today and not deferred until tomorrow.

Since optimal wellness is the goal, a total nutrition package must be indicated. Complete and balanced nutrition necessitates small, regular and varied meals - balanced for protein, carbohydrates and essential fats, low in refined foods, as well as salt and sugar. Raw, unprocessed organic foods are more desirable. These meals should then be supplemented daily to ensure an adequate supply of all the essential vitamins and minerals, especially anti-oxidants.

Finally, the hallmark of **Stem Cell Nutrition** must be emphasized.

That involves regular intake of stem cell enhancers that stimulate their release and other natural products to favor their circulation and migration. It completes the picture of a practical Wellness Lifestyle.

WELLNESS LIFESTYLE SUMMARY

- **No Smoking**
- **Managed Stress**
- **Positive Mental Attitude**
- **Moderate Exercise**
- **Adequate Rest/Sleep**
- **Complete and Balanced Nutrition including SUPPLEMENTATION**

So far, that's all as it should be. It's the expected lifestyle of health and wellness champions, generally recognized as the only responsible way to live. But in today's world, there is something more to add – something to make a winning difference. It is the defining characteristic of the modern **STEM CELL LIFESTYLE**. That's what this book is all about – the recent addition of **STEM CELL NUTRITION** – using edible natural products to promote and enhance the normal function of stem cells. That function - in which stem cells leave the bone marrow, traffick to tissues in need, then proliferate and differentiate to become cells of any particular tissue – represents

The Latest Breakthrough in the Wellness Revolution.

STEM CELL ENHANCERS Support Stem Cell	- **Release**
	- **Circulation**
	- **Migration**

With such a Stem Cell Lifestyle, each individual can choose to pursue optimal wellness and enjoy the best that life has to offer because.

The Take-Home Message

Everybody has stem cells; everybody uses stem cells; everybody uses stem cells everyday; stem cells work... and they work every time.

That is a good story to tell in our generation. It's a story in two parts. First, the normal **Natural Renewal System** of the body involves the release of those stem cells from the bone marrow. They then traffick to tissues in need where they migrate out, then proliferate and differentiate to become cells of each particular tissue, thereby providing an effective means for renewal and repair.

That's what nature does already!
That is stem cell physiology!

Second, dietary intervention through **Stem Cell Nutrition** is now available to enhance this intrinsic process in a mild but significant way, thereby making the promotion of optimal health and wellness available to all – **today**, not tomorrow or whenever there is visible light on the research horizon, through *Stem Cell Medicine*.

That's what you can do NOW
to support your own stem cell physiology!

That leaves us only to speculate about the Stem Cell Future. It's what the last chapter is all about ....

CHAPTER 12

The
STEM CELL
Future

The Stem Cell Future
is
UNPREDICTABLE

The pluripotent ability of Stem Cells makes all things possible biologically and therefore makes the future unpredictable. These cells are capable of doing anything we can conceive and even more...

"Prediction is difficult, especially if it's about the future."
-Neils Bohr, Danish physicist, philosopher

The Stem Cell Future
is
THERAPEUTIC

The great hope of Stem Cell Research is to use Stem Cells eventually as spare parts for the human body to rescue worn-out or diseased tissues at will...

"It is change, continuing change, inevitable change that is the dominant factor in society today. No sensible decision can be made any longer without taking into account not only the world as it is, but the world as it will be ... This in turn, means that ... everyone must take on a science fictional way of thinking."

- Isaac Asimov (1981), Russian born US author.

The Stem Cell Future
is
LIMITED

Each Stem Cell seems to have a mind of its own
controlled by its own molecular dictates.
Stem Cell Science seeks to understand that
mind in order to usurp its control.
Stem Cells will cooperate for sure, but we
must first condescend to their agenda...

*"Every science has for its basis a system of principles as fixed and
unalterable as those by which the universe is regulated and gov-
erned. Man cannot make principles; he can only discover them."*

- Thomas Paine, 18th century British-American political activist.

The Stem Cell Future
is
PROBLEMATIC

In order to use Stem Cells routinely - through medical intervention - for effective organ repair or replacement,at least two big challenges must be overcome: risk of rejection and fear of carcinogenesis...

"Life is not simply a series of exciting new ventures. The future is not always a whole new ball game. There tends to be unfinished business. One trails all sorts of things around with me, things that simply won't be got rid of."

- Anita Brookner (1989), British Novelist

The Stem Cell Future
is
SUBORDINATE

The best minds, the best ideas and the best biotechnology invented by man will never be an adequate substitute for the simplest and oldest spontaneous processes of nature, Stem Cell activity included...

Technological change defines the horizon of our material world as it shapes the limiting conditions of what is possible and whatever is barely imaginable. It erodes ... assumptions about the nature of our reality, the 'pattern' in which we dwell, and lays open new choices."

-Sloshana Zuboff (1988), US social scientist.

The Stem Cell Future
is
UNIVERSAL

Stem Cell Medicine can only hope to address the
needs of a tiny fraction of the human population.
Stem Cell Nutrition, on the other hand,
will always offer a benefit to all.
But each individual must still
make that choice...

*"Most of us are about as eager to change as we were to be born,
and go through our changes in a similar state of shock."*
- James Baldwin (1985), US author.

The Stem Cell Future
is
CONTROVERSIAL

Scientific Stem Cell research will continue to
pose moral and ethical challenges because the
science of certain types of stem cells
goes to the heart of what makes us human.
We cannot be detached or indifferent to
its implications...

*"Only man is not content to leave things as they are but must
always be changing them, and when he has done so, is seldom
satisfied with the result."*

– Elopeth Huxley, British author

The Stem Cell Future
is
HERE AND NOW

Stem Cell Medicine is all in the future – dependent on the progress of challenging research. Breakthroughs will come eventually ... but who knows when?

Stem Cell Nutrition is a solution for the present – dependent only on personal lifestyle choice.

"Everyone here has the sense that right now is one of those moments where we are influencing the future."

- Steve Jobs, US technology icon.

12-Point

SUMMARY OF PART IV

1. The Wellness Movement for the past forty years has been a response to four things: the industrialization of the food supply; persistent chronic disease despite the efforts of the high-tech medical establishment; disregard for all things natural and concomitant environmental abuse, and finally, a failure to recognize and support the integrity of the whole person.

2. Stem Cell (SC) Nutrition offers new possibilities for taking responsibility to practice illness prevention, and in a most natural way, it can influence the overall health of the whole person. As such, it is a new paradigm for wellness.

3. SC Nutrition is essentially not an invention but only a discovery of what nature provides to meet an intrinsic need. Since the normal renewal process involving adult stem cells helps to sustain health and optimize wellness, nature provides edible sources to enhance that innate physiological system.

4. To gain an understanding of stem cells in order to achieve control of their characteristics and function requires mammoth research efforts. Nature reveals such secrets only after long and arduous experimentation. But nature has always provided simple solutions in safe natural products that – like food – supply solutions to basic needs.

5. SC Medicine faces a daunting challenge. The routine application of stem cell therapy must overcome at least the prospects of rejection and the risk of tumor formation. Persistent research

will yield results some day, but in the meanwhile, SC Nutrition offers the opportunity for enhancing innate stem cells in a mild but meaningful way.

6.   SC Nutrition is a positive intervention, best understood and appreciated as a protector and preserver of life at its best and health in its most robust state. It is first and foremost, a form of primary prevention, without qualification.

7.   Medicine is practiced by the pursuit of definitive diagnosis and subsequent treatment of the same. SC Nutrition does not target particular organs or malfunctions, but rather, it empowers the body as a whole unit and helps the overall healing and renewal process.

8.   If SC Medicine is the next best hope for superlative break-throughs in curing disease (when that is the focus) in the future, then SC Nutrition is the best new strategy for opti-mizing health today.

9.   The Stem Cell Lifestyle is consistent with everything else we know about healthy living. That suggests no smoking, managed stress, positive mental attitude, moderate exercise, adequate rest/sleep, and finally, complete and balanced nutrition, including supplementation.

10.   SC Nutrition can make the winning difference to the typical wellness lifestyle. By ingesting stem cell enhancers, one can support overall stem cell physiology that includes the release, circulation and migration into needy tissues where they can effect renewal and repair.

11.   The Stem Cell Future is unpredictable, therapeutic, limited by nature, problematic, subordinate to nature and has

universal appeal, but – most important of all – it is here and now! SC Nutrition is a solution for the present, dependent only on personal lifestyle choice.

12. **Everybody has Stem Cells; everybody uses Stem Cells; everybody uses Stem Cells every day; Stem Cells work and ... they work every time. STEM CELL NUTRITION gives you a personal handle to enhance that important reality!**

Stem Cell-Based Therapies

As far as stem cells are concerned, it seems that for quite some time the media spotlight and public interest has been exclusively on cell-based therapies, including the promising 'miracles' of *regenerative medicine*. Now the public dreams of rebuilding spinal cords for victims of spinal cord injuries in wheelchairs, or arresting and reversing the slow painful degeneration of patients with serious neurological conditions like Alzheimer's, Parkinson's, or ALS (Lou Gehrig's disease). We can imagine restoring malfunctioning endocrine organs that lead to diabetes or Grave's or Addison's disease, or rescuing dying tissues that would result in cardiac or renal failure. What of reversing infertility on the one hand or slowing the aging process on the other? This is the new and promising revolutionary era of medicine that many now think is being ushered in on the horizon, thanks to stem cell research.

Having said all that, what real progress has been made to date? What have we learned, at least at the time of writing this brief review of the research into stem cell therapies? We'll now look at some of the promising areas.

We turn first to neurological illness because this area has been so much in the news and there are such prevalent cases of degenerative disease with rather hopeless and chronic suffering that weighs down many families. These illnesses provide the perfect storm for those

families because they combine 3 'P' factors. They occur with relatively high **prevalence**, with usually morbid **predicament** and with
generally poor **prognosis.**

As mentioned earlier, for many years it was standard dogma to
assume that the highly sophisticated neurons of the central nervous
system (CNS) were too specialized to be renewable[1]. In simple
terms, brain tissue could not be regenerated after birth. Then
researchers discovered in 2000 that adult neurogenesis (the formation of new neurons) was the result of proliferation and differentiation of stem cells residing in the brain[2,3]. Today neurogenesis is
well understood to develop from neural stem cells that locate along
the ventricles of the brain (that hold the cerebrospinal spinal fluid),
in a specific area called the hippocampus[4]. We now know that not
only can brain cells be replaced, but that phenomenon is in reality an
integral part of the natural renewal system whereby stem cells do
leave the bone marrow, migrate into the brain and become glial cells
(that form the scaffolding matrix) and actual brain neurons[5]. Such
migration of bone marrow stem cells into tissue could prove to be
important for any possible repair process in degenerative processes
(like Alzheimer's, Parkinson's and Multiple Sclerosis), as well as in
traumatic conditions (like spinal cord injury and stroke). Here's
what normally happens. When a brain injury occurs, neural stem
cells attracted by chemokine factors released from the injured area,
travel directly to the site of injury to begin effecting repair[5,6]. Also,
injection of adult stem cells directly into various parts of the nervous
system has shown some limited but promising clinical effects in several of these cases of CNS injury. There is no question today that
stem cells from the bone marrow have the capacity to become brain
cells[7,8].

Alzheimer's Disease

Up to 30 million people around the world suffer from this devastating illness with progressive, debilitating morbidity. Families suffer as a whole, just watching loved ones undergo helpless and hopeless personality changes with loss of memory, cognitive impairment and dementia often accompanied in the later stages by psychosis (loss of reality) and even aggressive behaviour. There is presently no effective treatment and therefore, clinical management is limited to nutritional support, physical safety and palliative care.

The root of this disorder is the malfunction and loss of some specific brain neurons that use acetylcholine as their neurotransmitter. These cells produce amyloid proteins that accumulate into characteristic plaques that further destroy brain tissue. Stem cell therapy, in principle, would seek to regenerate the so-called cholinergic neurons.

A few studies have been done using the injection of stem cells directly into the brain of laboratory animals. There has been only limited success related to change in clinical behaviours. The best results have used direct implantation of neural stem cells which were pretreated with genes that encode for neural growth factors. Following implantation, these cells develop in the brain and secrete their neural growth factors to trigger local neural stem cells to proliferate. The observed result in rats showed some improvement in both memory and learning cognition[9].

Another recent study used a different approach. They stimulated stem cell release from the bone marrow in mice by injecting G-CSF for five days and demonstrated that there was significant improvement in cognitive function, lasting up to three months[10].

These are yet early results in any possible stem cell treatment for Alzheimer's disease and pertain only to laboratory animals. As yet, there have not been any human trials of such therapy.

Parkinson's Disease

This disease can be considered essentially as a movement disorder. Like Alzheimer's, it is a progressive degenerative disease resulting from loss of neurons – but this time, using a different neurotransmitter called dopamine. These neurons are located in the characteristic region of the mid brain known as the striatum or *substantia nigra* (black substance). In medical schools, the symptoms of Parkinson's are often labelled by the acronym TRAP: Tremors, Rigidity, Akinesia (slow movement) and Postural disturbances. There may be some associated signs of cognitive change but oftentimes Parkinson patients remain quite mentally sharp and alert.

Some researchers reprogrammed adult mouse skin cells to generate dopamine- producing neurons and injected those into the brains of Parkinson rats[11]. They were able to demonstrate that the symptoms significantly improved.

Early attempts at the transplantation of fetal brain tissue that was rich in dopamine-producing neurons directly into the brain of a few Parkinsons patients did show some promise, because the transplanted cells not only survived, but appeared to revitalize the striatum functions for a few years[12,13]. But that fetal source was certainly controversial and clearly inadequate for any generalized therapeutic application. The same could be said for embryonic stem cells which also proved effective in primates with model Parkinson's[14]. Therefore, again we must look to adult stem cells for a possible feasible remedy.

Stem cells from the bone marrow and from human unbiblical cords have been transplanted directly into the brains of animal models with Parkinson's[15,16]. Those cells survived and differentiated into new neurons which migrated into the striatum specifically, unlike with control animals. Again they survived and significantly improved the motor skills of the affected animals. Similar results have been confirmed in humans[17].

There are still considerable challenges to be overcome before any stem cell therapy could become a probable widespread treatment/ solution for Parkinson patients. Manipulating stem cells - which includes isolating, culturing, maintaining, modifying, implanting and much more – can always pose significant risks and indeed possible complications with unforeseen and unintended consequences. In a 2006 study, for example, researchers first coaxed human embryonic stem cells to become dopaminergic neurons and then transplanted the latter into parkinsonion rats. The cells did significantly improve motor function, but when the rats' brains were examined after three months, they found many of the grafts contained groups of undifferentiated cells which had become cancerous[18]. These are the kinds of challenges that must be understood and addressed.

But there is hope. In one very recent study, researchers produced genetically altered skin cells to further study the effects of mutation in Parkinson's disease[19]. They reprogrammed skin cells from a patient with inherited PD and coaxed them to become diseased iPSC-derived nerve cells. They were able to correct the mutant gene in some of the iPS cells and then coax corrected iPS cells to become nerve cells too. These results allowed them to make useful comparisons between the diseased cells and the normal cells, to get a better handle on the underlying pathophysiology of Parkinson'sdisease.

Progress continues to be made.

Multiple Sclerosis

This is another neuro-degenerative condition that can lead to major physical dysfunction and sometimes cognitive loss as well. It pertains to the loss of the myelin insulating sheath that surrounds the nerve axons. Myelin speeds up nerve conduction and is a key factor in nerve control and body coordination. The typical presentation would be of an otherwise healthy young adult female, who shows neurological deficits (malfunction) in at least two areas, separated by space and time. Almost any neurological function can be affected. The disease tends to have a progressive course, sometimes with slow and steady decline, or at other times with alternating flare-ups or catastrophic downturn.

Myelin is a lipid layer made by specific cells – Schwann cells and oligodentroyctes – and the MS condition is believed to result from autoimmune attack on those cells. Cell-replacement therapy aims to use stem cells to replace those particular myelin- producing cells which in turn would replace the myelin sheaths and therefore restore adequate nerve function.

When stem cells are cultured in vitro in the presence of growth factors and compounds such as retinoic acid, they can differentiate into Schwann cells and oligodendrocytes that do produce myelin[20,21]. Using live animal models with demyelinated nerves, researchers showed that injection of GFP-labelled bone marrow stem cells into their spinal cords did remyelinate their spinal nerves[22]. Using the standard Walling Tract Test as a measure, the animals showed significant improvement after such treatment[23].

These promising animal models gave rise to early human trials[24]. A select group of 19 MS patients in Italy, with fairly advanced disease, were treated with their own bone marrow stem cells by spinal cord injection. All of them showed stabilization and sometimes improvement in their symptoms. This procedure has also been confirmed elsewhere.

An alternate approach using direct injection of bone marrow stem cells into the blood has also produced effective regeneration of the spinal cord(25-27). In this case, the stem cells must migrate to the affected areas inside the spinal column. And that they do. But this method required twice as many stem cells for comparable results. In either case, the degree of success was directly proportional to the number of bone marrow stem cells injected.

All these results indicate that stem cell therapy is a very promising therapeutic intervention in the case of MS. The somewhat effective nerve repair in the study cited earlier, has led to symptom improvement and therefore offers hope for many patients around the world. Yet problems do remain.

Spinal Cord Injury

In the United States alone the incidence of spinal cord injury (SCI) has been estimated to be about 40 cases per million per year, or around 12,000 cases per year. There are some 300 – 500,000 individuals living with SCI, the large majority of whom are males. The condition typically results from car and diving accidents, falls, violence and sports injuries, occurring at an average age around 40. Depending on where the spinal cord and nerve roots are damaged, the symptoms can vary widely, from incontinence and chronic pain to paralysis (notably hemiplegia and quadriplegia). The loss of function can be partial or complete. Currently no effective treatments are known and medical management is essentially supportive.

This is one area that has captured the imagination of the general public. Once the potential value of stem cells in the regeneration of cells (and therefore tissues) was exposed by the media, there has been wide speculation. What if we could develop a new biotechnology, for example, to repair the (usually) local site of damage to the spinal nerves and restore function? What potential that would afford the thousands of SCI victims, offering what could be dramatic improvements in their quality of life and restoring hope for their caring families. But unfortunately, there still has been no major breakthrough to enable clinicians to offer any substantial treatments.

Regardless of the statistics, it is fair and encouraging to report that some very early progress is being made. At least we know that injection of bone marrow stem cells (BMSC) directly into the spinal cord of paraplegic rats significantly improved their gait within weeks[28]. New bundles of nerve tissue appeared at the site of injury to form an effective bridge across the nerve lesions. These benefits were realized when injection of the BMSC was done as late as three months after the SCI[29].

In other experiments, microscopic examination of rat spinal cords after injection with human neural stem cells (HSC) demonstrated that the HSC had not only become nerve cells, but they formed working connections with the rat spinal and nerve cells[30]. Other HSC become supporting cells that covered parts of the injured spinal cord with new myelin.

Other researchers demonstrated that using G-CSF to stimulate the release of stem cells from the bone marrow, again in rats and one week after rendering them paraplegic, resulted in gradual improvement in locomotion, muscle reflexes and hind limb sensitivity over the course of a few weeks, when compared to normal controls. There was obvious formation of new nerve cells and white matter at the site of injury[31].

In most of these experiments on rats, there appears to be a critical period of time following injury when the intervention with stem cells is most effective. It may turn out to be true, that the potential value of stem cells in this kind of regenerative treatment, at least with SCI, may be limited to those patients who can be treated soon after injury and unfortunately not be so hopeful for the victims of injuries when treatment is delayed. Only time will tell.

We have a long way to go before any miraculous cures for SCI can be achieved but someone has wisely observed that 'the greatest journey on earth always begins with the next step.' As we mentioned before, early progress in the treatment of SCI in laboratory animals was promising enough for the USFDA to approve in 2009 the only real human trial of stem cell therapy to date, notably on the treatment of SCI. However, the company behind the trial made a decision to discontinue that trial in 2011, reportedly due to purely 'financial reasons'[32].

Stroke

A stroke is the common term for what is clinically referred to as a cerebrovascular accident, leading to rapid loss of brain function due to a disturbance in the blood supply to the brain. Classically, there are two types: one due to ischemia (inadequate blood flow) usually resulting from a blood clot, the other due to haemorrhage in the brain. The net result is that cells die and the affected areas of the brain cannot function adequately. This could manifest as one or more deficits in movement, vision, speech or cognition and other symptoms. It constitutes a medical emergency when symptoms like these appear, since acute intervention could, by all accounts, limit the damage and alter prognosis. Several risk factors should always heighten suspicion including increased age, a history of high blood pressure, previous stroke or TIA (a warning of stroke), diabetes, elevated cholesterol, smoking and irregular heartbeat. Stroke is serious business and it rates among the leading causes of death around the world. It is also the source of much chronic disability and suffering, affecting entire families.

Some consequences of stroke are irreversible despite the best in medical management. Rehabilitation is often very helpful in restoring some levels of function, depending on the severity of the event itself and the speed and efficiency of the initial emergency response.

Here is another area where the public has real expectation for some kind of breakthrough with stem cells. There is hope of restoration and repair of damaged cells, especially with all the media reports of miraculous potential, including the exaggerated properties of stem cells. Yet stroke prevention represents the best hope for practical intervention.

Research is being actively pursued to explore the potential value of stem cell therapy for stroke victims at least as an ultimate goal. Early results showed that injection of some particular brain-committed stem cells in adult rats, four weeks after a stroke, led to improved motor and cognitive responses[33,34]. That led to a small scale clinical trial with 12 human stroke patients. The positive results observed confirmed that this approach could be feasible, effective and relatively safe[35]. But unfortunately in that initial case, those cells injected were of cancerous origin. Others have since used embryonic stem cells with promising results too,[36] but the ethical problems and supposedly high risk of induced cancer still remained. But researchers are beginning to get a handle on this risk. For example, culture methods have been developed to cause human neural stem cells to become mature neurons, with no residual undesirable and undifferentiated cells[37]. Transplants of these cells in rats produced no signs of tumors, at least up to the two months of observation, while improving function in those rats that had suffered a stroke.

There is some better news. When bone marrow stem cells were injected into the brain after stroke, at least in animals, they did migrate to the site of injury and improved blood flow there[38]. These cells are known to enhance the secretion of growth factors in the brain, which helps to facilitate the entire recovery process. In fact, the injury itself seems to trigger the release of cytokines that enhance stem cell release from the bone marrow which can triple in the first week after an injury. Recovery appeared to correlate directly with the number of these bone marrow stem cells. The improved function recovery seen in rats, using human stem cells, can then be accounted for by the formation of new brain cells in addition to factors that promote blood flow and intrinsic healing of the brain.

Although tissue stem cells are generally able to replace injured cells following normal wear and tear, the same spontaneous renewal process does not seem adequate to repair or correct more severe organ damage, as seen in stroke victims. This reflects their inability to proliferate within the tissues. Researchers have isolated neural stem cells from humans and injected then with a virus carrying v-myc, a factor known to be important in self-renewal, while combining tetracycline as a regulator in the culture media[39]. This generated large numbers of stem cells which when transplanted in mice with stroke, migrated to affected areas, differentiated there into new neurons and glia, and showed even better improvement of stroke symptoms.

And that's all exogenous. Not surprisingly, studies that use G-CSF to mobilize bone marrow stem cells endogenously in rats, also demonstrated impressive functional improvement within a few weeks[40]. The evidence all suggests that when brain injury takes place, increased stem cell release is first stimulated from the bone marrow. Then circulating stem cells selectively migrate to the areas affected and in several ways help to support the functional recovery of the damaged tissue[41]. Naturally, increasing the number of stem cells trafficking to the brain should only enhance recovery and favour a much better prognosis. If only this could all prove to be safe and even more effective in humans in years to come. To that end, research continues.

Before we leave the area of the nervous system, two more conditions ought to be addressed even in this limited review of stem cell therapies in general. One pertains to a leading cause of visual limitations, especially in later life, and the other to a slow and quite debilitating nerve disease first made popular by the famous baseball player, Lou Gehrig.

Vision Changes

Perhaps one of the most distressing physical conditions is to lose one's eyesight. The most common disease that leads to decline and even loss of vision is age-related macular degeneration (ARMD). Unlike cataracts which can easily be cured by replacing the relatively opaque natural lens of the eye with a new clear intraocular lens implant, ARMD has no known effective cure. Here, the neurons and particularly the light-sensitive cells (photoreceptors) in the retina (screen) at the back of the eye, lose their ability to function adequately. In a word, cells die at the back of the eye and the renewed hope for therapy is that stem cells can somehow come to the rescue. Can they get there and then differentiate into new functional retinal cells with responsive rods and cones to facilitate improvement in vision?

We do know that stem cells from the bone marrow have been injected into the eyes of rats and they were able to get into the retina and differentiate to become active retinal cells that carry electrical impulses[42]. In fact, using human embryonic stem cells (hESCs), scientists have derived retinal pigment epithelium (RPE) [43]. RPE is a supporting layer of cells that helps to protect and enable the function of the rods and cones in the retina. When rats with a genetic eye disease similar to ARMD were injected with the RPE cells, there was clear improvement in visual acuity[44]. Some British scientists also report other results with RPE derived from induced pluripotent stem cells[45]. They found a clear benefit in preserving retinal integrity and vision, but only if given before degeneration began. By what mechanism you wonder? The authors suggested that either the transplanted cells attract the host's inflammatory response (with phagocytes removing debris in place of the lost RPE function) or they may have a neuroprotective effect. In a very recent and limited Phase 1 trial, some other researchers injected hESC-derived RPE into the eye of one patient with ARMD to test the safety and tolerability of this method of therapy. They followed up with one other patient, this time with Stargardt disease (an inherited MD seen earlier in life). In both cases, the treatment was well tolerated and both patients experienced improved vision in the treated eye[46]. This is very preliminary, of course, but such results, again, are quite promising.

Once more, and not surprisingly, stem cells from the bone marrow have also been demonstrated to migrate to the eyes on their own, to do the same thing. Animal models suggest that within hours of retinal damage, those injured cells secrete SDF-1 and other growth factors to enhance release and trafficking of stem cells from the bone marrow,[47] just as we have detailed in general, earlier. Any therapy that exploits intrinsic or endogenous stem cells from the bone marrow would certainly offer great advantages .... Let's therefore hope for more success in that direction.

Lou Gehrig's Disease

Lou Gehrig was a superstar, hall-of-fame first baseman and batting champion for the New York Yankees. He had a durability that earned him the nickname 'The Iron Horse', but his distinguished career was cut short at age 36 when he was stricken with a degenerative neurological disease that doctors call amylotrophic lateral sclerosis (ALS). Two years later it eventually took his life, as it does for almost all its victims.

ALS is characterized by rapidly progressive weakness, muscle atrophy (wasting) and fasciculations (twitching), muscle spasticity and difficulties associated with speaking, swallowing and worst of all, breathing. To say that 'it is not nice' is a euphemistic understatement. There is no certain cause but many suggested ones. What we do know for sure is that the upper and lower motor neurons in the central nervous system die off.

Treatment for ALS is now unfortunately limited to symptomatic relief and finally palliative care. The incidence of the ALS condition is fortunately quite low – limited to just one or two people per 100,000 each year. Each case is somewhat different and so the prognosis varies. One cannot but refer to probably the most famous ALS patient since Lou Gehrig, namely the Cambridge Theoretical Physicist and Cosmologist, Stephen Hawking. He was born in 1942, diagnosed at age 21 and still remains today as one of the most brilliant minds on planet earth. Surprise!

Getting back to stem cells and ALS, it is not surprising that research has been directed at ALS in exploring possibilities of repairing (or restoring function at least) or even replacing the affected CNS motor neurons. In at least one study where paralysed rats were used as ALS models, researchers transplanted pluripotent cells derived from human embryonic germ cells and demonstrated that it was possible to partially restore the ability to move[48]. The transplanted cells migrated into the rats' spinal cords and prevented existing host neurons from dying. The cells seemed to restore mobility by secreting factors that promote the re-growth of connections between in-growing nerves and motor neurons. Again, such results are very preliminary but at least they point in the right direction of hope.

Therefore, hope remains as work in the area continues.

Heart Disease

We now turn from the devastating chronic conditions and diseases of the nervous system to the number one killer in developed countries, which is heart disease.

Stem cells have created the exceedingly high level of excitement because they have the potential value of treating 'the big ones' since they offer the possibility of repairing and restoring the types of damaged and even dead cells that for so long had been considered helplessly and hopelessly irreversible and irreplaceable. Heart disease is just like that. Inadequate blood supply to the heart muscle (usually from blocked coronary arteries) causes insufficient oxygen to sustain the muscle cells and the tissue cells begin to die. That could lead to angina on the low end, a heart attack (or myocardial infarction) in the middle or sudden death at the extreme. Over one million heart attacks occur every year in the United States and about 60% of victims survive, usually with scarring of the heart muscle that again, had been considered irreversible. So what might be the possible role of stem cells in heart disease? Could stem cells do something to reduce the incidence and severity of heart attacks in the first place? And then could they do anything to help restore scarred heart muscle to improve function and ameliorate the prognosis for those surviving victims who must wrestle with all the challenges of cardiac rehabilitation?

The good news answers are both Yes! and Yes!

Recent evidence has pointed to the fact that cardiac cells are actually regenerating constantly[49-51]. There is a continuous stream of circulating stem cells migrating from the bone marrow and into the heart. These numbers would be enough to maintain the estimated loss of some approximately seven million heart cells per year. But with chronic heart disease, even a 10-fold increase in normal proliferation still proves to be insufficient to restore the damaged heart muscle after an acute attack[52]. That's the natural state of affairs.

In one study, female mice were injected with GFP-labelled stem cells from the bone marrow of male mice[53-55]. The injections were made directly into the heart muscle wall and adjacent to the infarcted (scarred) area. On examination, a new band of heart muscle could be observed across the area of previously scarred heart tissue. That new cardiac muscle was clearly derived from the injected cells and showed many functional characteristic ties of normal cardiac muscle cells. There were also signs of smooth muscle cells forming new blood vessels within the regenerated heart muscle. These were also shown to originate from the injected stem cells.

However, it is useful to note that in studies like this, the regenerated heart muscle tissue did not fully integrate structurally with the viable portion that survived intact. The 'repaired' portions seemed to form a secondary structure which did not completely harmonize with the remainder of the heart during the cardiac cycle of contraction and relaxation.

Results like this led to a few Phase 1 trials with actual survivors of heart attacks. For example, 10 patients had standard treatment for their heart attacks and then soon had bone marrow stem cells infused via a balloon catheter right into the artery supplying blood to the area of infarction[52]. Three months later, their heart function was compared to another matched group of 10 heart attack patients, with very positive results. There was less scarring, increased muscle wall contraction, better emptying of the heart in systole and an increased blood supply to the area. It has since been confirmed that these hopeful improvements are only seen when the stem cell intervention is made relatively soon after a heart attack. Attempts to ameliorate heart muscle structure and function in patients with old myocardial infarction have not been quite as successful[56].

It is worth noting that researchers have already demonstrated that both human embryonic stem cells (hESC) and induced pluripotent stem cells (IPSC) have been used to derive cardiac muscle cells. So in principle, one could imagine using a patient's own skin cells, reprogramming them to derive iPSCs and cardiac muscle cells for repairing their heart muscle[57]. This again negates issues of immuno-suppression and possible rejection which must always be considered in cases of transplantation.

Again, it's one thing to inject stem cells exogenously (from outside), it's quite another to enhance the normal migration of stem cells from the bone marrow to increase trafficking to the heart to help repair heart muscle and restore function. This has also been demonstrated after inducing a heart attack in animals and then injecting cytokines like G-CSF and SCF over the course of a few days[53,54]. This led to increased migration of stem cells to the injury site and proliferation and differentiation there, leading to new cardiac muscle tissue and also new blood vessel formation around the affected ventricle. Red blood cells could be detected microscopically. Only 17% of all the untreated animals in the study survived, and they showed residual cardiomyopathy (floppy hearts) and compromised blood circulation. But of those treated, 73% survived and did so with much better cardiac function and improved blood circulation.

Similar studies on humans showed quite variable results depending on the different protocols used[58-62]. One might expect results to vary with different researchers looking at similar therapies involving enhanced migration of bone marrow stem cells to treat heart attacks, but under different conditions. No clear consensus may immediately emerge. Yet despite controversy, one must always look for indications of hope. And the net conclusions must be that this general approach could be successfully used sometime in the future to treat heart attacks soon after they occur. In fact, a meta-analysis of seven such studies with a total patient count at 364, and a second one reviewing eight studies and 385 patients, both led to the conclusion that after heart attacks, treatment of patients with G-CSF does improve left ventricular ejection fraction (at least one good indication of heart performance) as long as the treatment is administered early[63]. But several other general indicators of cardiac health were not so definitively changed so the jury is really still out on the effectiveness of this therapy.

Diabetes

From the big questions of possible stem cell therapy in heart disease, we turn next to another big one: diabetes. It's big and getting even bigger, especially in North America. Almost one and a half million Americans now suffer with this disease.

Diabetes is the common term used to reference what is medically classified as *diabetes mellitus* (DM). (The alternate condition diabetes insipidus is relatively rare and won't be considered here). DM is a metabolic condition in which sugar (glucose) in the blood is unable to get into the cells of the body, due to a decline in insulin function. In insulin-dependent DM (Type 1) the B-cells of the pancreas make insufficient insulin, whereas in non-insulin dependent DM (Type 2) there is insulin available but its action is less effective.

Blood glucose is the key energy source in the body, and when cells are deficient, they essentially starve and die. At the same time, the high glucose levels in the blood attacks proteins like haemoglobin which can lead to major problems also. The clinical consequences of diabetes mellitus can be severe. It affects the microcirculation that can lead to heart disease, kidney failure and blindness. It can cause peripheral vascular disease and poor wound healing that sometimes leads to amputation. It may also destroy nerves.

The common symptoms to alert an individual to possible diabetes might include: increased urination and excessive thirst, unexplained weight loss, blurring of vision, weakness and lethargy. Confirmation by simple tests in a doctor's office can readily pin down the diagnosis. Once that happens, management of the condition is key. Since insulin was discovered in Toronto in 1921 by Banting and Best, the curse of the disease has been lifted but still no real cure has been found. In addition to the important diet control, weight loss and exercise, oral medications that potentiate the action of insulin have gone a long way in helping Type 2 patients regulate blood sugar levels and therefore improve their quality of life and overall prognosis.

The so-called Type 1 diabetes is more commonly seen at a younger age. It is generally believed to be an auto-immune disease - in other words, the patient's own immune system attacks the B-cells of the pancreas causing a decline in insulin production. When it falls to a significant low (usually when some 60-80% of the B-cells are knocked out) the symptoms of insufficient insulin become more pronounced. Hopefully a clear diagnosis is made and treatment with regular insulin injections becomes mandatory and usually quite effective. In the later stages of Type 2 diabetes, it is not uncommon to increase insulin by adding injections to the oral medications to gain more effective control of blood sugar levels.

It is now clear that stem cells from the bone marrow can differentiate into functional insulin-producing pancreatic B-cells[64]. When this was done in vitro and then injected into diabetic rats, blood glucose levels were observed to fall[65]. More importantly, stimulating the release of stem cells from the bone marrow in human subjects, led to lower blood glucose levels, the formation of new blood vessels in the pancreas and in some cases, it was possible to effectively stop the prescribed use of insulin[66]. That's very promising.

Using the same green fluorescent protein (GFP) we discussed earlier, researchers were able to demonstrate unequivocally in mice, that the stimulation of bone marrow stem cells allowed them to migrate to the pancreas to become insulin-producing cells and actively participate in forming new blood vessels to further support the pancreas[67,68]. Surprisingly, when bone marrow stem cells themselves were injected directly into the pancreas, other researchers observed no similar effects[69]. Apparently, the *natural mobilization* of the bone marrow stem cells appears somehow to be essential in this case.

CONCLUSION

Despite all the promising advances just described, as researchers continue to exploit the possibilities of stem cell-therapy, it is still apparent that no widespread application of all that stem cell science is imminent. It would therefore be unwise to anticipate some dramatic development that will provide any miraculous cures through Stem Cell Medicine in the near future, since major hurdles remain. There is so much that we still do not know or have a good handle on. But we are making significant strides.

However, at the same time, the benefits of **Stem Cell Nutrition** are now available to support the normal daily renewal process that promotes optimal wellness. That's great news today for anyone choosing to take personal responsibility for their health status, focusing on prevention as they exploit natural alternatives and target the protection and improvement of their whole person. It's a recipe worth pursuing as part of a Stem Cell Lifestyle that is definitely worth living.

That's the Amazing Power of STEM CELL NUTRITION!

REFERENCES

PART I

Chapter 1

1. Maximov A (1969) Lecture to Hematol Soc of Berlin: "The Lymphocyte as Common Stem Cell of the different Blood Elements during Embryonic Development and in the Post-Fetal Life of Mammals."

2. Till JE, McCulloch EA (1961), *Radiat Res,* 4:213-222

3. Thomson JA et al. (1998), *Science,* 282(5391):1145-7

4. Shanblott MJ, Axelman J, Littlefield W (2001), *Proc Natl AcadSci USA,* 98(1):113-8

5. Perin L et al. (2008), *Methods Cell Biol,* 86:85-99

6. Yamanaha S et al. (2006), *Cell,*126:1-14

7. Brighton CT, Hunt RM, *J Bone and Joint Surg,* 73A(6):832-847

8. Brighton CT, Hunt RM, *J Orthop Trauma,* 11(4):244-253

9. Bossolasco P et al. (2005), *Exp Neurol,* 193(2):312-325

10. Sato Y et al. (2005), *Blood,* 106(2):756-763

11. Rojas M et al. (2005), Am J Resp : *Cell Mol Biol,* 33(2):145-152

12. Chen LB, Jiang XB, Yang L (2004), *World J Gastroenterol,* 10(2):3016-20

13. Nagaya N et al. (2005), *Circulation,* 112(8):1128-35

14. Bongso A, Richards M (2004), *Best Pract Res Clin Obstet Gynaecol,* 18(6):827-42

15. Chan-Ling T et al. (2006), *Am J Pathol,* 168(3):1031-44

16. Orlic D et al. (2001), *Proc Natl Acad Sci,* USA, 98(18):10344-9

17. Cui HF, Bai ZL (2003), *World J Gastroenterol,* 9(10):2274-7

18. (a) Jang YY et al. (2004), *Nature Cell Biol,* 6(6):532-9
    (b) Lagasse E et al. (2000), *Nat Med,* 6(11):1229-34

19. Sigurjonsson OE (2005), *PNAS,* 102(14):5227-32

20. Krause DS (2001), *Cell,* 105:369-377

21. Zuba-Surma EK (2008), *J Cell Mol Med,* 12(1):292-303

22. (a) Woodbury D et al. (2000), *J Neurosci Res,* 61:364-370
    (b) Sanchez-Ramos JR (2002), *ibid.,* 69:880-893

23. Schwartz RE et al. (2002), *J Clin Invest,* 109:1291-1302

24. Jiang Y et al. (2002), **Nature**, 418(6893):41-49

25. Shimomura O, Johnson F, Saiga Y (1962), *J Cell Comp Physiol,* 59(3):223-239

26. (a) Ikawa M et al. (1995), *Dev Growth Differ,* 37:455-9

    (b) Kawakami N et al. (1999), *Immunol Lett,* 70:165-171

    (c) Ramiro AR et al. (1998), *Hum Gene Ther,* 9:1103-9

    (d) Parsons DA et al. (1998), *Nat Med,* 4:1201-5

    (e) Ono K et al. (1999), *Biophys Res Commun,* 262:610-4

    (f) Wu YP et al (2000), *Am J Pathol,* 156:1849-54

Chapter 2

1. Jensen GS, Drapeau C (2002), *Med Hypotheses,* 59(4):422-8

2. See Ref. 26 for Chapter 1

3. Krause DS et al. (2001), *Cell,* 105:369-377

4. Bensinger W et al. (1996), *Bone Marrow Transplant,* 17:S19-21

5. Cottler-Fox et al. (2003), *Amer Hematol Soc – Hematol Educ Program* 419-437

6. Fibbe WE et al. (1999), *Ann NY Acad Sci,* 872:71-82

7. Mannello F et al. (2006), *Stem Cells,* 24(3):475-481

8. Robbins SL et al. (1998), *Pathological Basis of Disease*, WB Saunders Co., Phila. Publ.

9. James JL, Carter AM, Chemley LW (2012), *Placenta,* 33(5):327-334

10. Kohn LA et al. (2012), *Nat Immunol,* 13(10):963-971

11. Frenette PS, Weiss L (2000), *Blood,* 96(7):2460-8

12. Jensen et al. (2007), *Cardiovasc Revasc Med,* 8(3):189-202

13. Graf L, Heimfeld S, Torok-Storb B (2001), *Biol Blood Marrow Transplant,* 7:486-494

14. Mohle R et al. (1993), J Hematother, 2(4):483-9

15. Powell TM et al. (2005), *Arterioscler Thromb Vasc Biol,* 25(2):296-301

16. Aiuti A et al. (1997), *J Exp Med,* 185(1):111-120

17. Peled A et al. (2000), *Blood,* 95(11):3289-96

18. Gerhartz HH, Fliedner TM (1980), *Exp Hematol,* 8 (suppl 2):209-218

19. Kucia M et al. (2004), *Blood Cells Mol Dis,* 32(1):52-57

20.   Neuss S et al. (2004), *Stem Cells*, 22:405-414

21.   Voermans C et al. (2000), *ibid.*, 18(6):435-443

22.   Peled A et al. (1999), *J Clin Invest*, 104(9):1199-1211

23.   Janowska-Wieczorek A (2000), *Exp Haematol*, 28:1274-85

24.   Askari AT et al. (2003), *Lancet*, 362(9385):697-703

25.   Ratajczak MZ et al. (2003), *Cell*, 21(3):363-371

26.   Hatch HM et al. (2002), *Cloning Stem Cells*, 4(4):339-351

27.   Kollet O et al. (2003), *J Clin Invest*, 112(2):160-9

28.   Bagri A et al. (2002), *Development*, 129:4249-60

29.   Lazarini F et al. (2003), *Glia*, 42:139-148

30.   Zou Y et al. (1998), *Nature*, 393:595-599

31.   Schrader AJ et al. (2002), *Br J Cancer*, 86(8):1250-6

32.   Wojakowski W et al. (2004), *Circulation*, 110(20):3213-20

33.   Abbott JD (2004), *ibid.*, 110(21):3300-5

34.   Takahishi T et al. (1999), *Nat Med*, 5(4):434-8

35.   Iwaguro H et al. (2002), *Circulation*, 105:732-738

36.   Kollet O et al. (2003), *J Clin Invest*, 112(2):160-9

37.   Ratajczak MZ et al. (2004), *Leukemia*, 18:29-40

38.   Swenson ES et al. (2008), *Liver Int*, 28(3):308-318

39.   Tomoda H, Aoki N (2003), *Clin Cardiol*, 26(10):455-457

40.   (a) Werner N et al. (2007), *Basic Res Cardiol*, 102(6):565-571

       (b) Werner N et al. (2005), *N Engl J Med*, 353(10):999-1007

41.   Michaud SE et al. (2006), *Atherosclerosis*, 187(2):423-432

42.   (a) Chan HK, Oza AM, Siu LL (2003), *Clin Cancer Res*, 9:10-19

       (b) Kirsch C, Eckert GP, Mueller WE (2003), *Biochem Pharmocol*,
       65:843-856

43.   Jin FY et al. (2006), *Zhonghua Yi Xue Za Zhi*, 86(42):2966-70

44.   Avigdor A et al. (2004), *Blood*, 103(8):2981-9

45.   Friedl P et al. (1997), *Cancer Res*, 57:2061-70

46.   Bonavia R et al. (2003), *Toxicol Lett*, 139:181-9

47.   Broxmeyer HE et al. (2003), *J Leukoc Biol*, 73:630-8

48.   Lataillade JJ et al. (2002), *Blood*, 99:1117-29

49.   Hwang JH et al. (2006), *Stem Cells Dev*, 15(2):260-8

50.   Arsenijevic Y et al. (2001), *J Neurosci*, 21(18):7194-7202

51. Deasy BM et al. (2002), *Stem Cells*, 20(1):50-60

52. Mishra SK et al. (2006), *Development*, 133(4):675-684

53. (a) Shytle DR et al. (2010), *Medical Science Monitor,* 16(1): BR1-5. PMID 20037479

     (b) Bickford PC et al. (2006), *Stem Cells Dev*, 15(1):118-123

54. Mias C et al. (2008), *Stem Cells*, 26(7):1749-57

55. Camargo FD et al. (2003), *Nat Med,* 9(12):1520-7

56. Ferrari G et al. (1998), *Science,* 279(5356):1528-30

57. (a) Okamoto R et al. (2002), *Nat Med ,* 8:1011-17

     (b) Okamoto R,Watanabe M (2003), *Trends Mol Med*, 9:286-290

58. (a) Lee KD et al. (2004), Hepatology, 40:1275-84

     (b) Sco MJ et al. (2005) *Biochem Biophs Res Commun*, 328:258-264

59. (a) Sordi V et al. (2005), *Blood*, 106:419-427

     (b) Seeberger KL et al. (2006), *Lab Invest*, 86:141-153

60. (a) Pereira RF et al. (1995), *Proc Natl Acad Sci USA*, 92:4857-61

     (b) Pereira RF et al. (1998), *ibid.*, 95:1142-7

61. Eglitis MA et al. (1997), *ibid.*, 9:4080-5

62. Tomita M et al. (2002), *Stem Cells,* 20(4):279-283

63. Jackson KA et al. (2001), *J Clin Invest,* 107(11):1395-1402

64. Orlic D et al. (2001), *Proc Natl Acad Sci USA*, 98(18):10344-9

65. Terada N et al. (2002), *Nature*, 416(6880):542-5

66. Vassilopoulos G, Wang PR, Russell DW (2003), *ibid.*, 422(6934):901-4

67. Spus JL et al. (2003), *Proc Natl Acad Sci USA*, 100(5):2397-2402

68. Wurmser AE, Gage FH (2002), *Nature*, 416(6880):485-7

69. Bonde S. et al. (2010), FASEB *Journal*, 24(2), 364-373

70. Jang YY et al. (2004), *Nat Cell Biol*, 6(6):532-9

71. Rustom A et al. (2004), *Science*, 303(5660):1007-10

72. Thiese ND et al. (2000), *Hepatology*, 32(1):11-16

73. Thiele J et al. (2004), *Transplantation*, 77(12):1902-5

74. Quaini F et al.(2002), *N Engl J Med*, 346(1):5-15

75. Laflamme MA et al. (2002), *Circ Res*, 90(6):634-640

76. Korbling M et al. (2002), *N Engl J Med*, 346(10):738-746

77. Poulsom R et al. (2001), *J Pathol*, 195(2):229-235

78. Mezey E et al. (2003), *Proc Natl Acad Sci USA,* 100:1364-9

Chapter 3

1.   Stein R, *Washington Post (2011),* November 14

2.   Lanza R et al. (2006), *Nature,* 444(7118):481-5

3.   Rigoutsos I, Loring J, Wei C (2010), *Genome Research,*

4.   Lander ES et al. (2006), *Cell,* 125(2):315-326

5.   Young RA et al. (2006), *ibid.,* 125(2):301-313

6.   Boyer LA et al. (2006), *Nature,* 441:349-353

7.   Sun Y et al. (2007), *Proc Natl Acad Sci USA,* 104(34):13821-6

8.   Jaenisch R et al. (2004), *Genes and Development,* 18:1875-85

9.   Smith A, Jaenisch R et al. (2006), *Stem Cells,* 24:2007-13

10.   Yang X, Cheng T et al. (2006), *Nature Genetics,* 38:1323-28

11.   Jaenisch R et al. (2006), *Proc Natl Acad Sci USA,* 103:933-8

12.   Daley GQ (2007), *Science,* 315:482-8

13.   Janus JD (2007), *Cloning Stem Cells,* 9(3):432-449

14.   Yamanaka S et al. (2006), *Cell,* 126:1-14

15.   Yamanaka S (2007), *Cell,* 131:861-872

16.   Thomson J et al. (2007), *Science,* 318:1917-20

17.   (a) Jaenisch R et al. (2007), *Nature,* 448(7151):318-324

      (b) Yamanaka S (2007), *ibid.,* 448(7151):313-317

18.   Melton et al. (2008), *ibid.,* 455(7213):627-663

19.   Scholer H et al. (2008), *ibid.,* 454:646-650

20.   Hochedlinger K (2008), *Cell Stem Cell,* 2(3):230-240

21.   Cibelli JB et al. (2009), *Stem Cell Dev,* 19(8):1221-9

22.   Nagy A et al. (2009), *Nature,* 458(7239):766-770

23.   Woltjen K et al., *ibid.,* 458(7239):771-5

24.   Rossi DJ (2010), *Cell Stem Cell,* 7:1-13

25.   Daley GQ, Feinberg AP et al. (2009), *Nat Genet,* 41(12):1350-3

26.   Benvenistry N et al (2010), *Cell Stem Cell,* 7:521-531

27.   Bhatia M et al. (2010), *Nature,* 468:521-6

28.   Hochedlinger K et al. (2010), *Nat Biotech,* 28(8):848-55

29.   Xu Y et al. (2011), *Nature,* 474:212-6

30.   Reproductive Biomedicine OnLine, 10:105-110

31.   Eggan K et al. (2008), *Science,* 321(5893), 1218-21

32.   Hochedlinger K et al. (2008), *Cell,* 134(5):877-886

33. Svendsen C et al. (2008), *Nature*, 457(7227):277-280

34. Muotri AR et al. (2010), *Cell*, 143:527-539

35. Dolmetsch R et al. (2011), *Nat Med,* 17:1657-62

36. Gage F et al. (2011), *Nature,* 473:221-5

37. Thomson J et al (2011), *PNAS*, 108:6537-42

PART II

Chapter 4

1. Nutritional Evaluation of Food Processing, 2nd Ed (1975), Harris RS, Karmas E, eds, AVI Publishing, Westport, CT

2. Holmberg SD et al. (1984), *N Engl J Med*, 311(10):617-622

3. Modern Nutrition in Health and Disease, 6th Ed (1980), Goodhart RS, Shils ME, eds,Lea and Febiger, Phila, PA, Publ.

4. Gahche J et al. (2011), Dietary Suppl Use Among US Adults. CDC-NCHS Data Brief No.61

5. Shaw GM et al. (1995), *Epidemiology*, 6(3):219-226

6. Daley S et al. (1997), *Lancet,* 350(9092):1666-9

7. Ross AC et al. (2011), Dietary Reference Intakes for Ca and Vit D, Wash DC: *Natl Acad Press* p. 435. ISBN 0-309-16394-3

8. Wagner CL, Greer FR (2008), *Pediatrics*, 122:1142-52

9. Cranney C et al. (2007), AHRQ Rockville, MD, Publication No. 07-E013

10. Reiffel JA, McDonald A (2006), *Amer J Cardiol*, 98(4A):50-60

11. Herbaut C (2006), *Revue medicale de Bruxelles*, 27(4):S355-360

12. (a) Logan AC et al. (2004), *Lipids in Health and Disease*, 3(1):25
     (b) Sublette ME et al. (2011), *J Clin Psych*, 72(12):1577-84

13. Barnes P et al. (2004), CDC Advance Data Report No. 343

14. Laing C et al. (2006), *Lancet*, 368(9532):338

15. DaSilva EJ et al. (2002), *Electronic J Biotech*, 5(1), April 15

16. Fabricant DS, Farnsworth NR (2001), *Environ Health Perspect,* 109(Suppl 1):69-75

17. USFDA/CFSAN, A Food Labelling Guide: Appendix C, Health Claims, April 2008

18. Cooper K (1994), Antioxidant Revolution, *Thomas Nelson Publ.*

19. Somersall AC (1999), Breakthrough in Cell Defense, *NWG*, Toronto

20. Gutman J (1998), Glutathione, Gutman and Schettini, Montreal, Publ.

21. (a) Bounous G, Gold P (1991), *Clin Invest Med,* 14:296-309

    (b) Bounous G, Batist G, Gold P (1989), *ibid.,* 12:154-161

22. Lands LC, Grey VL, Smountas AA (1999), *J Appl Physiol,* 87:1381-5

23. Corder R et al. (2006), *Nature,* 444(7119):566

24. Baur JA, Sinclair DA (2006), *Nat Rev Drug Discov,* 5(6):493-506

Chapter 5

1. Jensen GS, Drapeau C (2002), *Medical Hypotheses,* 59(4):422-8

2. Pugh N et al. (2000), *Planta Med,* 67:737-742

3. Jensen GS et al. (2000), *J Amer Neutr Assoc,* 2(3):50-58

4. Hart AN et al. (2007), *J Med Food,* 10(3):435-441

5. Romay C et al. (1998), *Inflamm Res,* 47:36-41

6. Sabelli ... et al. (1996), *J Neuropsych Clin Neurosci,* 8:168-171

7. Consumer Reports Magazine (1999), pp. 44-48

8. *Ibid.,* May 2004

9. Mazey E et al. (2000), *Science,* 290:1779-82

10. Jensen GS et al. (2007), *Cardiovasc Revasc Med,* 8:189-202

11. Krause DS et al. (2001), *Cell,* 105:369-377

12. Frenette PS, Weiss L (2000), *Blood,* 96(7):2460-8

Chapter 6

1. (a) Zhao M et al. (2003), *PNAS,* 100(13):7925-30

    (b) Tomita M et al. (2002), *Stem Cells,* 20(4):279-283

    (c) Kawada H et al. (2006), *Circulation,* 113(5):701-710

2. (a) Ince H et al. (2005), *ibid.,* 112(20):3097-3106

    (b) Orlic D, Hill JM, Arai AE (2002), *Circ Res,* 91(12):1092-1102

    (c) Orlic D et al. (2001), *PNAS,* 98(18):10344-9

3. Kollet O et al. (2003), *J Clin Invest,* 112(2):160-9

4. Herrerra MB et al. (2004), *Int J Mol Med,* 14(6):1035-41

5. (a) Ianus A et al. (2003), *J Clin Invest,* 111(6):843-850

    (b) Lee RH et al. (2006), *PNAS,* 103(46):17438-43

6. (a) Rojas M et al. (2005), *Am J Respir Cell Mol Biol,* 33(2):145-152

    (b) Yamada M et al.(2004), *J Immunol,* 172(2):1266-72

7. (a) Mansilla E et al. (2006), *Transplant Proc,* 38(3):967-9

    (b) Borue X et al. (2004), *Am J Pathol,* 165(5):1767-72

8. (a) Bozlar M et al. (2005), *Saudi Med J,* 26(8):1250-4

    (b) Burt RK et al. (2004), *Arthritis Rheum,* 50(8):2466-70

9. Cumashi A et al. (2007), *Glycobiology,* 17:541-542

10. Tissot B et al. (2003), *Biochem Bophys Acta,* 1651:5-16

11. (a) Thring TS et al. (2009), *Complement Alt Med,* 9:27

    (b) Senni K et al. (2006), *Arch Biochem Biophys,* 445:56-64

12. Meyers SP et al. (2010), *Biologics,* 4:33-44

13. Cashman JD (2011), *J Surg Res,* 171(2):495-503

14. Hayaski S et al. (2008), *Eur J Pharmocol,* 580:380-4

15. Hemmingson J et al. (2006), *J Appl Phycol,* 18:185-193

16. Irhimeh MR, Fitton JH, Lowenthal RM (2007), *Exp Haematol,* 35:989-994

17. (a) Sweeney EA et al. (2000), *Proc Natl Acad Sci USA,* 97:6544-9

    (b) Fermas S et al. (2008), *Glycobiology,* 18:1054-64

18. Mavier P et al. (2004), *Am J Pathol,* 163:1969-76

19. Chung HJ et al. (2010), *Phytother Res,* 24:1078-83

20. Li N, Zhang Q, Song J (2005), *Food Chem Toxicol,* 43:421-6

21. (a) Li Shuang LV et al. (2006), *J Food Lipids,* 13(2):131-144

    (b) Zheng B et al. (1990), *Gerontology Magazine,* 10(5):306

    (c) Gao-Qin HE et al. (1987), *Chinese Med Pharmocol Clin Applic,* 3(4):41

    (d) Kimura Y et al. (1983), *Planta Med,* 49(1):51

22. Jung KA et al. (2011), *Gut Liver,* 5(4):493-9

23. Diabetes Mellitus : A Fundamental and Clinical Text, 3rd Edit (2004). Lippincott, Williams and Wilkins, Phila, PA, Publ., LeRoith D, Taylor SI, Olefsy JM eds.

24. (a) Grimble RF (1994), *New Horiz,* 2(2):175-185

    (b) Rodriguez-Porcel M et al. (2004), *Hypertension,* 43(2):493-6

    (c) Copp SW et al. (2009), *Exp Physiol,* 94(9):961-971

    (d) Chai Siah Ku et al. (2013), *J Medic Food,* 16(2):103-111

25. Pais E et al. (2006), *Clin Hemorheology and Microcirc,* 35:139-142

26. Fujita M et al (1995), *Biol Pharm Bull,* 18(10):1387-91

27.   Unpublished Results. Available on line @ www.stemtech.com

28.   Parker EM , Cubeddu LX (1998), *J Pharmocol Exp Ther,* 245:199-210

29.   Paterson IA (1993), *Neurochem Res*, 18:1329-36

30.   Shannon et al. (1982), *J Pharmocol Exp Ther*, 223:190-6

31.   Szabo et al. (2001), *Brit J Sports Med*, 35:342-3

32.   Sabelli HC et al. (1976) (www.ncbi.nlm.nih.gov/pubmed/9160)

33.   Sabelli H et al. (1978), *Biochem Pharmocol,* 27:1707-11

34.   Baker GB et al. (1991), *Biol Psych*, 29(1):15-32

35.   Grimsby J et al. (1997), *Nat Genetics*, 17:206-210

36.   Sabelli H et al. (1996), *J Neuropsych Clin Neurosci*, 8:168-171

37.   Jensen GS et al. (2000), *JANA*, 2(3):50-58

38.   Hart AN et al (2007), *J Med Food*, 10(3):435-441

39.   Pugh N et al. (2001), *Planta Med,* 67:737-742

40.   Romay Ch et al. (2003), *Current Protein and Peptide Science*, 4:207-216

41.   Romay Ch et al. (1998), *Inflamm Res,* 47:36-41

42.   Atanasiu RL et al. (!998), *Mol Cell Biochem,* 189:127-135

43.   Bhat VB, Madyastha KM (2000), *Biochem Biophys Res Comm,* 275:20-25

44.   Romay Ch., Gonzalez R (2000), *J Pharm Pharmocol*, 52:367-8

45.   (a) Spillert Ch et al. (1987), *Agents Actions*, 21:297-8

        (b) Halliwell B.... (1990), ... Rad Res Comm, 9:1-32

46.   Romay Ch, Ledon N, Gonzales R (1998), *Inflamm Res,* 47:334-8

47.   Opas EE, Bonney RJ,Humes JL (1985), *J Invert Dermatol,* 84:253-6

48.   Kushak RI et al. (2000), JANA, 2(3):59-64

PART III

Chapter 7

1.   Harrison M (2008), Edible Seaweeds around the British Isles. Ref Wikipedia/Edible Seaweed

2.   Thomas D (2002), Seaweeds, Natural History Museum, London. ISBN 0-565009175-1

3.   Fitton JH et al. (2002), *BMC Complement Alter Med*, 2:11

4.   Hu T, Dan Liu, Yan Chen, Jun Wu, Wang S (2010), *Intl J Biol Macromol,* 46(2):193-8

5.   Maeda H et al. (2005), *Biochem Biopys Res Comm*, 332(2):392-7

6.   Hehemann JH et al. (2010), *Nature*, 464(7290):908-912

7.   Johnston HW et al. (1970), *Tuatara,*18(1): 'Edible Algae of Fresh and Brackish Water'

8.   Farrar WV (1966), *Nature,* 211(5047):341-2

9.   Nemikawa S (1906), *Bull Coll Agric, Tokyo Univ*, 7:123-4

10.   Lee YK (1997), *J Appl Phycol,* 9:403-411

11.   Ayehunie S et al. (1998), J AIDS, 18(1), 7-12

12.   Barmejo-Bescos P et al. (2008), *Toxicology In Vitro*, 22(6):1496-1502

13.   Qishan P et al. (1989), *Toxic Letters,* 48:165-9

14.   Khan M et al. (2005), *Phytotherapy Res,* 19(2):1030-7

15.   Wang Y et al. (2005), *Exp Neuro*, 193(1):75-84

16.   Gemma C et al. (2002), *J Neurosci*, 22(14):6114-20

17.   Kulshreshtha A et al. (2008), *Curr Pharm Biotech,* 9(5):400-5

18.   ALSUntangled No.9: Blue-green Algae (Spirulina) as a treatment for ALS, ALS, 12(2):153-5

19.   Chen LL et al. (2005), *J Central South Univ* (MedSci), 309(1):96-98

20.   Simpore J et al. (2005), *Annals Nutr and Metab,* 49:373-380

21.   Mao TK et al. (2005), *J Medic Food*, 8(1):27-30

22.   Torres-Duran PV et al. (2007), *Lipids Health Dis*, 6:33

23.   Lu HK et al. (2006), *Europ J Appl Physiol,* 98(2):220-6

24   Chamorro-Cevallos G et al. (2008), 'Toxicologic Studies and Antitoxic Properties of Spirulina`in``Spirulina in Human Nutrition and Health` (CRC Press)

25.   Robb-Nicholson C (2006), *Harvard Women's Health,* 8

26.   Belasco W. (1997), *Technol and Culture*, 38(3):608-634

27.   Shim J-Y et al. (2008), *J Medic Food*, 11(3):479-485

28.   Blas-Valdivia V et al. (2010), *J Appl Phyco*, 23:53-58

29.   Merchant RE, Andre CA (2001), *Alt Ther in Health and Med*, 7(3):79-91

30.   Carmichael WW, Drapeau C, Anderson DM (2000), *J Appl Phycol,* 12:585-595

31.   (a) Jensen GS et al. (2000), *JANA*, 2(3):50-58

      (b) Pugh N, Pasca DS (2001), *Phytomedicine*, 8(6):445-453

      (c) Pugh N et al. (2001), *Planta Med,* 67:737-742

32.   Romay C et al. (1998), *Inflamm Res*, 47:36-41

33.   (a) Hanson GR et al. (2005), `Drugs and Society`, 9th Edit., *James & Bartlett, Publ.*

        (b) Sabelli HC et al. (1978), *Biochem Pharmocol*, 27(13):1707-11

34.   Jensen GS et al. (2007), *Cardiovasc Revasc Med*, 8(3):189-202

Chapter 8

1.   Carmichael WW, Drapeau C, Anderson DM (2000), *J Appl Phycology,* 12:585-595

2.   US Patent Applic Pub No. US2010/0147782 A1, June 17, 2010. Assignee: Desert Lake Tech

3.   US Patent No. 7,651,690 B2 Dated Jan 26, 2010. Assignee: Desert Lake Tech

Chapter 9

1.   Carmichael WW (1997),'The Cyanotoxins', Adv in Bot Res, Callow JA ed, *Acad Press*,pp 211-56

2.   Carmichael WW, Drapeau C, Anderson DM (2000), *J Appl Phycology*, 12:585-595

3.   Chu FS, Huang X, Wei RO (1990), *J Assoc Analyt Chem*, 73: 451-6

4.   An JS, Carmichael WW (1994), *Toxicology,* 32:1495-1507

5.   (a) Scallan E et al. (2011), *Emerg Inf Dis,* 17(1):16-22

        (b) Strom S (Jan 4, 2013), *New York Times*

6.   Dirikolu L et al. (2010), *Nutr Diet Suppl*, 2:125-135

7.   Dirikolu L et al. (2011), *ibid.*, 3:19-30

8.   Drapeau C et al. (2009), *Anticancer Research*, 29:443-8

9.   Liu Y et al. (2000), *J Appl Phycology*, 12:125-130

10.   Jensen GS et al. (2000), *J Amer Nutr Assoc*, 2:50-58

PART IV

Chapter 10

1.   (a) Vasa M et al. (2001), *Circ Res*, 89(1):E1-7

        (b) Werner N et al. (2005), *N Engl J Med*, 353(10):999-1007

2.   Marchesi C et al. (2008), *PLoS ONE*, 3(5):e2218

3.   Junhui Z et al. (2008), *Respir Med*, 102(7):1073-9

4.   (a) Herbrig K et al. (2006), *Ann Rheum Dis*, 65(2):157-163

        (b) Grisar J et al. (2005), *Circulation*, 111(2):204-211

5.   Zhu J et al. (2006), *Arch Med Res*, 37(4):484-9

6.   Westerweel PE et al. (2007), *Ann Rheum Dis*, 66(7):865-870

7.   Eizawa T et al. (2003), *Curr Med Res Opin*, 19(7):627-633

8.   Lee ST et al. (2008), *Neurology*, 70(17):1510-7

9.   Antarr D (2008), Abstract Mtg of the ISSCR, Philadelphia, Penn.

10.   School of Public Health, Harvard University, Boston, Mass.

11.   Danaei G et al. (2009), *PLoS Med*, 6((4)

Chapter 11

1.   Takashi U (2008), *Amer J Hypertension*, 21(11):1203-9

2.   Laurent GJ (1982), *Biochem J*, 206:535-544

3.   Rennard SI, Togo S, Holz O (2006), *Proc Am Thorac Soc*, 3(8):703-8

4.   Nyunoya T et al. (2006), *Am J Respir:Cell Mol Biol*, 35(6):681-8

5.   Wang H et al. (2001), *ibid.*, 25(6):772-9

6.   Miglino N et al. (2012), *Europ Respir J*, 39(3):705-711

7.   Nakamura Y et al. (1995), *Am J Respir:Crit Care Med*, 151(5):1497-1503

8.   Lin S et al. (2007), *Proc Ann Mtg of the ISSR*, p.127

9.   Ockene IS, Miller NH (1997), *Circulation*, 96:3243-47

10.   McVeigh GE et al. (1996), *Am J Cardiol*, 78:668-672

11.   Schachinger V , Britten MB, Zeiker AM (2000), *Circulation*, 101:1899-1906

12.   Moreno H Jr., et al. (1998), *Am J Physiol*, 275:H1040-45

13.   (a) Gill M et al. (2001), *Circ Res*, 88:167-174

        (b) Tateishi-Yuyama E et al. (2002), *Lancet*, 360:427-435

        (c) Shintani S et al. (2001), *Circulation*, 103:2776-9

14.   Takashi T et al. (1999), *Nat Med*, 5:434-438

15.   (a) Michaud SE et al. (2006), *Atherosclerosis*, 187(2):423-432

        (b) Kondo T et al. (2004), Arterioscler Thromb Vasc Biol, 24:1442-7

16.   The US Surgeon General's Report (2004) : The Health Consequences of Smoking

17.   Tran BT, Halperin A, Chien JW (2011), Biol Blood Marrow Transplant,

17(7):1004-11

18.   Liu XD et al. (2001), *J Lab Clin Med*, 137(3):208-9

19.   O'Keefe RJ et al. (2008), presented at Ann Mtg Orthop Res Soc, San Francisco

20.   Hitoshi S et al. (2006), *Proc Ann Mtg of the ISSCR*, p.103

21.   Saito T et al. (1997), *Surg Today,* 27(7):627-631

22.   Levite M (2008), *Curr Opin Pharmocol*, 8(4):460-471

23.   Ben-Eliyahu S et al. (1990), *Behav Neurosci*, 104(1):75-91

24.   De la Fuente M, Delgado M, Gomariz R (1996), *Adv Neuroimmunol*, 6(1):75-91

25.   Beresford L et al. (2004), *Immunology*, 111(1):118-125

26.   Katayama Y et al. (2006), *Cell,* 124(2):407-421

27.   Bonsignore MR et al. (2002), *J Appl Physiol,* 93(5):1691-7

28.   (a) Morici G et al. (2005), *Am J Physiol:*Regul Integr Comp Physiol, 289(5):R1496-1503

       (b) Schmidt A et al. (2007), *Brit J Sports Med*, 43(3):195-198

29.   Stout CI et al. (2007), *Amer Surg*, 73(11):1106-10

30.   Yarrington A, Mehta P (1998), *Pediatr Transplant*, 2(1):51-55

31.   Haldar C, Haussler D, Gupta D (1992), *J Pineal Res,* 12(2):79-83

32.   (a) Jiang HW, Ling JQ, Gong QM (2008), *J. Endod,* 34(11):1351-4

       (b) Garg R et al. (2008), *Catheter Cardiovasc Interv,* 72(2):205-9

33.   (a) Pais E et al. (2006), *Clin Hemorheol and Microcirc,* 35:139-142

       (b) Fujita M et al. (1995), *Biol Pharm Bull,* 18(10):1387-91

34.   Bickford PC et al. (2006), *Stem Cell Dev,* 15(1):118-123

Appendix

1.   Cajal SR, May RT (1959), Degeneration and Regeneration of the Nervous System. New York, NY. *Hafner* p.750

2.   Momma S, Johansson CB, Friesen J (2000), *Curr Opin Neurobiol*, 10:45-49

3.   Singh-Roy N et al. (2000), *Nat Med*, 6:271-7

4.   Rietze R, Poulin P, Weiss S (2000), *J Comp Neurol*, 427:397-408

5.   (a) Kopen GC, Prockop DJ, Phinney DG (1999), *PNAS*, 96:10711-6

      (b) Aarum J et al. (2003), *ibid.,* 100(26):15983-8

6. Hoehn M et al. (2002), *ibid.*, 99(25):16267-72

7. Sanchez-Ramos JR et al. (2002), *J Neurosci Res*, 69(6):880-93

8. Dezawa M et al. (2005), *Curr Neuropharmocol*, 3(4):257-266

9. Wu S et al. (2008), *Pathobiology,* 75(3):186-194

10. Tsai KJ et al. (2007), *J Exp Med*, 204(6):1273-80

11. Jaenisch R et al. (2008), *Proc Natl Acad Sci USA*, 105(15):5856-61

12. Lindvall O, Kokaia Z, Martinez-Serrano (2004), *Nat Med*, 10:542-550

13. Piccini P et al. (1999), *Nat Neurosci,* 2(12):1137-40

14. Takayi Y et al. (2005), *J Clin Invest,* 115(1):102-9

15. Weiss ML et al. (2006), *Stem Cells*, 24(3):781-792

16. Fu YS et al. (2006), ibid., 24(1):115-124

17. Levesque M, Neuman T (2002), *Amer Assoc of Neurol Surg,* Ann Mtg Abstract #702

18. Goldman S et al. (2006), *Nat Med*, 12:1259-68

19. Jaenisch R et al. (2011), *Cell,* 146:318-331

20. Tohill M, Terenghi G (2004), *J Exp Med*, 204(6):1273-80

21. Dezawa M et al. (2001), *Eur J Neurosci*, 14:1771-6

22. Akiyama Y, Radtke C, Kocsis JD (2002), *J Neurosci*, 22(15):6623-30

23. Cuevas P et al. (2002), *Neural Res*, 24:634-8

24. Saccardi R et al. (2005), *Blood*, 105:2601-7

25. Inome M et al. (2003), *Glia*, 44(2):111-8

26. Pluchino S et al. (2003), *Nature,* 422(6933):688-694

27. Su L et al. (2006), *Int J Haematol*, 84(3):276-281

28. Hofstetter CP et al. (2002), *PNAS*, 99(4):2199-2204

29. Zurita M, Vaquero J (2004), *Neuroreport*, 15(7):1105-8

30. Anderson AJ et al. (2005), *Proc Natl Acad Sci* USA, 102:14069-74

31. Urdzikova L et al. (2006), *J Neorotrauma*, 23(9):1379-91

32. Stein R, Washington Post (2011), November 14

33. Nishinott H, Borlongan CV (2000), *Prog Brain Res*, 127:461-76

34. Borlongan CV, Hess DC (2006), *CMAJ*, 174(7):954-5

35. Nelson PJ et al. (2002), *Am J Pathol*, 160:1201-6

36. Jin K et al. (2005), *Neurobiol Dis*, 18(2):366-374

37. Steinberg GK et al. (2008), *PLoS ONE*, 3(2):e1644

38. Pavlichenko N et al. (2008), *Brain Res*, 1233:203-213

39. Kim SU, Snyder E (2011), *Proc Natl Acad Sci* USA, 108:4876-81

40. Shyu WC et al. (2004), *Circulation,* 110(13):1847-54

41. Six I et al. (2003), *Eur J Pharmocol,* 458(3):327-8

42. Tomita M et al. (2002), *Stem Cells,* 20(4):279-283

43. Lanza R et al. (2004), *Cloning and Stem Cells,* 6:217-245

44. Lanza R et al. (2006), *ibid.,* 8:189-199

45. Carr et al. (2009), *PLoS One,* 4(12): e-8152

46. Schwartz S et al (2012), *Lancet,* 379:713-720

47. Li Y et al. (2006), *Invest Ophthalmol Vis Sci,* 47(4):1646-52

48. Gearhart JD, Rothstein JD et al. (2003), *J Neurosci,* 23:5131-40

49. Kajstura J et al. (1998), *Proc Natl Acad Sci USA,* 95:8801-5

50. Soonpaa MH, Field LJ (1998), *Am Heart Assoc J,* 83:15-26

51. Beltrami AP et al. (2001), *N Engl J Med,* 344:1750-7

52. Schwartz Y, Kornowski R (2003), *Heart Fail Rev,* 8(3):237-245

53. Orlic D et al. (2001), *Nature* (London), 410:701-5

54. Orlic D et al. (2001), *Proc Natl Acad Sci* USA, 98(18):10344-9

55. Orlic D et al. (2001), *Pediatric Transplant,* 7(Suppl 3):86-88

56. Kang HJ et al. (2006), *Circulation,* 114(suppl 1):1145-51

57. Zhang J et al. (2009), *Circ Res,* 104(4): e30-41

58. Inu H et al. (2005), *Circulation,* 112(suppl 1):I73-80

59. Seiler C et al. (2001), *ibid.,* 104:2012-7

60. Ellis SG et al. (2006), *Am Heart Assoc J,* 152(6):1051.e9-14

61. Zohlnhofer D et al. (2008), *JACC,* 51:1429-37

62. Ripa RS, Kastrup J (2008), *Exp Hematol,* 36(6):681-6

63. Kang S et al. (2007), *Clin Ther,* 29(11):2406-18

64. Lu P et al. (2007), *Diabetes Res Clin Pract,* 78(1):1-7

65. Chen LB et al. (2004), *World J Gastroenterol,* 10(20):3016-20

66. Voltarelli JC et al. (2007), *JAMA,* 297(14):1568-76

67. Matthews V et al. (2004), *Diabetes,* 53(1):91-98

68. Gao X et al. (2008), *Biochem Biophys Res Commun,* 371(1):132-7

69. Hasegawa Y et al. (2007), *Endocrinology,* 148(5):2006-15

To Order Additional Copies of

The Amazing Power of
STEM CELL NUTRITION

VISIT US AT:

www.stemcellnutrition.com

Made in the USA
Lexington, KY
12 June 2013